Life Hacked

A Comprehensive Guide to Immortality

by

Jacob Clifton

Life Hacked: A Comprehensive Guide to Immortality

Table of Contents

Introduction: The Quest for Everlasting Life

Imagine a world where the ticking clock no longer spells the end, where the fine lines etched on faces become badges of wisdom, not decay. Ever since the first breaths of ancient civilizations, humanity has been enthralled by the concept of immortality: a state of existence where the final curtain call is indefinitely postponed. And it's not just a tale spun by mystics and dreamers; from the rigorous labs of cutting-edge science to the mind-body connection honed by millennia of tradition, the quest for everlasting life is the ultimate human journey.

It's a winding path, peppered with the myths of the ancients, promising a glimpse into the psyche of our ancestors: their values, their fears, and their overwhelming desire to conquer mortality. But before delving deep into the labyrinth of immortality, let's take a moment to understand the lay of the land. This introduction doesn't just set the table; it lays out the map for the intrepid traveler determined to understand the power and promise of life without an end.

What zips through your neurons when you think about living forever? The bliss of endless years or the weight of ceaseless existence? We'll venture into that philosophical den, scrutinize the ethical scaffolds that prop up our society, and we might just dabble in the murky waters of morality. But that's just the crest of the wave. Deep beneath the surface, an ocean of scientific endeavors rages — from the mysteries of our very cells to the digital horizons that might harbor our minds for eternity.

What's more, there's an unmistakable hum in the zeitgeist: the body as a temple, the mind as a universe, and the spirit as an uncharted dimension. It's about priming the pump, fueling the engine with the finest nutrition, marrying meditation with muscular movement, syncing the symphony of our consciousness with the physical vessel it calls home.

And let's not forget the tech. Oh, the tech! Silicon and circuits potentially ushering in the next chapter of human evolution, where biological boundaries blur, and horizons stretch into the infinite. But as we stare into the promising abyss of eternity, we mustn't lose sight of the rocky shores — the risks, the ethical quagmires, the societal shudder that might come with a world brimming with ageless souls.

So let's embark on this odyssey together. It's not just about tagging along for a marathon read (although, make no mistake, we're in this for the long run). It's about the fiery core of what makes us human: the relentless pulse in our veins that drives us to explore the unknown and pushes us to extend not just our lifespans but the quality of the lives we lead. It's about redefining the essence of life, death, and the ethereal in-between — a quest not just for more time, but for an era of enriched existence.

Welcome to the beginning. Welcome to the wonder, the science, the maybes and the certainties. Welcome to the melting pot of extant knowledge and the future that beckons with the promise of youth eternal. This is the quest for everlasting life, and it starts now.

Chapter 1: Introduction to Immortality

Peering into the abyss of time, it's hard not to be mesmerized by the echo of an age-old question bouncing off the walls of human consciousness – what if we could outlive the stars. Let's dive headfirst into the eternal enigma of immortality. It's a concept that's been dancing through the dreams of humanity since the first storyteller spun tales beneath the moon's glow. Across the broad tapestry of history, every culture under the sun has whispered its own secrets about defying the reaper's persistent call. We've yearned for the Philosopher's Stone, the Fountain of Youth, for ambrosia that would set our souls ablaze with unending life. Yet, amid the labyrinth of tales and quests, immortal life's true essence remains as elusive as the wisp of a dream at dawn's first light. This chapter isn't just about the whimsy of what-ifs; it's the starting block of a marathon that winds through the annals of time – a profound quest to understand the riddle that has tickled and tormented philosophers, pharaohs, and physicists alike. Here is where we set the stage, tracing the footsteps of an odyssey that is as much about the journey as it is about the destination – a primer on humanity's pursuit of the infinite, a story without an end.

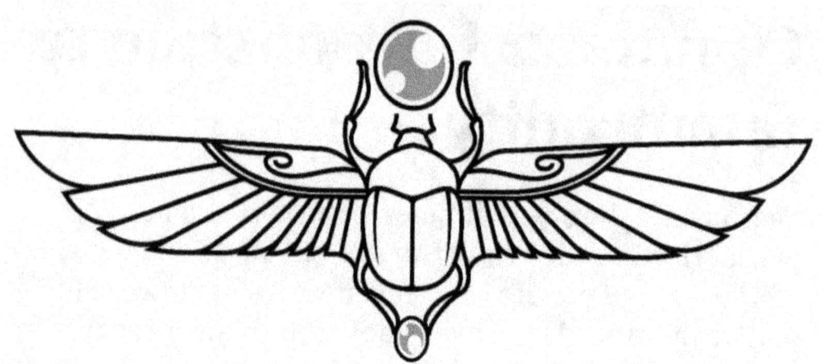

Exploring the concept of immortality

Let's dive into the deep end, where the waters of immortality swirl with mystery and fascination. It's a concept that has tickled the edges of human curiosity since we first became aware of our own mortality. What if the body could outlast the wear and tear of time? What if the essence of humanity could endure forever? It's more than just not aging; it's about transcending the very notion of death.

At its core, immortality is as elusive as it is alluring. We're talking about a state of being that defies the only certainty of existence: life concludes. But what if it didn't have to? That's where the mind begins to race, and possibilities start to unfurl like an infinite canvas. Can we cheat the inevitable, or is it folly to try? This isn't an exercise in futility; it's a call to push the boundaries of what we believe is achievable.

Throughout history, stories and legends hint at a longing to break free from the chains of mortality. Alchemists sought their Philosopher's Stone, rumored to grant immortality. Myths speak of gods with the power to bestow eternal life. There's a seduction in these narratives, a whispered promise that taps into our primal desire to persist eternally. But let's be honest, immortality as folklore is one thing; facing the actual implications of achieving it is quite another.

Isn't there a paradox in seeking something so contrary to life as we know it? Life, in its essence, is a series of cycles: birth, growth, decay, and death. To eliminate one part of the cycle is to invite questions we might not be ready to answer. Yet here we are, attempting to keep the conversation on immortality earnest and grounded, even as our imagination wants to run wild.

So, where are we on this journey? Pausing to consider the state of our current existence, it's enough to wonder if we're even built for immortality. Physically, perhaps the human machine can be tweaked, reshaped, and maintained. There's intrigue in the thought of a body that can regenerate itself indefinitely, a heart that beats without end. Yet, mentally and emotionally—are we equipped to handle the weight of endless tomorrows?

Delving into the role of our consciousness in this quest, we poke at the nebulous interface of self-awareness. Is immortality merely a biological continuity, or does it also imply the perpetual stream of thoughts, memories, and experiences that form the tapestry of an individual's essence? Immortality might not just be fighting the decaying of flesh and bone, but also preserving the spark that makes each of us uniquely ourselves, potentially forever.

Imagine for a moment the application of immortality within our lives. The relationships we build, the knowledge we acquire, the experiences we cherish—how would they morph if the end point were erased? Would we love differently, learn ceaselessly, and savor moments with an intensity unknown to those bounded by lifespans? It brings into play a richness to life and interactions that bears exploring, a level of depth where timing isn't everything because there's always more.

However, the pursuit of immortality begs a slew of ethical and existential quandaries. What happens when the natural order is disrupted? Do resources stretch to accommodate an immortal populace? Can Earth sustain its children who refuse to leave the nest? We look to the promise of immortality with starry eyes, but the harsh glare of logistics can't be ignored. How does society adapt to minimize the fallout of a world where death takes a backseat?

But the biggest question in our exploration might just be this—why do we seek immortality? Is it a fear of non-existence, a hunger for endless opportunity, or something else entirely? It's these deeper, sometimes dark corners of our psyche that become illuminated when we dare to face the prospect of eternal life. Toying with immortality is as much about understanding the bounds of human psyche as it is about conquering the biological constraints of our bodies.

In the end, pondering immortality isn't just about the ambition to live indefinitely. It's also about the here and now, how we choose to spend our days, and what it means to be alive in this moment. Immortality might be a grand horizon, sparkling on the edge of human potential, but what truly matters is how its pursuit shapes us today. As we muse on what it means to exist indefinitely, let's embrace the richness of the conversation and the transformation it beckons within us all.

Historical and cultural perspectives on immortality

When we let our thoughts wander through time, touching the ancient sands of Egypt or the mystical lands of China, we often stumble across humanity's age-old obsession with immortality. Think about it, the Egyptians weren't just playing around with mummies and pyramids for fun—they were neck-deep in the business of forever. They believed in an afterlife so strongly that they spent their whole lives (and deaths) prepping for it.

But let's jump over to the Greeks, shall we? The ever-fascinating folks who tossed around tales of ambrosia and the gods like they were discussing the weather. For them, immortality was a feast, accessible only to the divine residents of Olympus. And yet, there was this relentless, burning desire in humans to grab a seat at that table. It speaks volumes, doesn't it? That hunger for eternity was never just about surviving—it was about finding the ultimate table of belonging, the apex of achievement.

Move a bit forward in time, and you've got the alchemists—now there's a group that could talk your ear off about immortality. They were the OG mad scientists, mixing up elixirs of life and hunting down the Philosopher's Stone. It wasn't just a Rowling invention, folks—it was a genuine quest for the mightiest of makeovers: the immortal kind. And it wasn't just about living longer but transforming the soul, turning base human metal into gold.

Now, let's not forget the East, blending spirituality with immortality like they invented the smoothie. Buddhism and Hinduism talk about the cycle of life, death, and rebirth, hinting that maybe immortality is a game of quality, not quantity. It's the level-up from mere survival into enlightenment, an unending journey of the soul that might just loop us back to the very essence of existence.

But buckle up—actually, scratch that; let's take a leisurely stroll through the Middle Ages. That's where we find alchemy's lamppost-lit streets morphing into the Fountain of Youth. Explorers burned through their maps seeking this liquid legend, convinced that somewhere out there, there was a puddle of water that could undo the creakiness of their bones. It was the physical incarnation of hope, liquid 'just-one-more-day-please' for the taking.

Across the pond, you can't talk immortality without tipping your hat to the indigenous legends, where the concept gets painted with broader strokes. Immortality was woven into the fabric of the world, a part of an intricate tapestry that included animals, plants, and celestial pachinko machines. To them, it was less about personal forever and more about the seamless cycle of life—everything connected in a balance that hummed with eternity.

Fast forward to the Renaissance, and enter the vampires. OK, so they might not have been strutting around Florence, but they were in the stories, slipping through the shadows as undying symbols of the allure and fear entangled in immortality. They whispered a tempting question: what price would you pay for a never-ending night?

And now, in our modern tale-spinning society, we've got sci-fi turning the telescope on immortality. It's no longer ethereal. It's become something to engineer, a bug in the system to fix, a disease to cure. It's a sci-fi writer's dream and a philosopher's contemplative playground. With longer lifespans within our grasp—thanks to leaps in medicine and technology—the once-distant dream of immortality might just be another thing to add to the to-do list.

From fountain-hunting to genetic twiddling, each era and each culture has sculpted its own vision of immortality. They've painted it with the brushes of their values, their fears, their envies, and their highest hopes. And while the methods have morphed and the stories have shifted, the theme stays as stubborn as a stain: we're fascinated by the idea of cheating the clock, of laughing in the face of time and saying, "Not today, Chronos, not today."

It's this epic, sprawling history of humanity's chase after immortality that sets the stage for our current musings. We're the latest in a long line of forever-chasers, and our place in this lineage is both humbling and exhilarating. As we stand on the shoulders of these past cultures, grasping at our own place in the eternity conversation, it becomes clear that immortality isn't just a concept—it's a cultural tapestry, rich with the colors of every age that has dared to dream of a life beyond the final breath.

The Quest for Eternal Life Throughout Human History

Imagine standing on the banks of a river that flows through time. Dip your fingers in the water, and you touch the dreams of countless generations, all reaching for that elusive current called 'immortality.' It's a pull as ancient as the pyramids, an obsession that's older than the written word. The quest for eternal life is not just a chapter in history; it's the entire saga of humanity, etched deeply into our collective psyche.

Across every era and civilization, the yearning for life without end has taken center stage. From the Epic of Gilgamesh, where a hero scours the earth for a plant that can restore youth, to the pharaohs interred with spells to guide their souls to everlasting life, our ancestors weren't just riffing on a theme—they were painstakingly composing an opus to their disdain for the final curtain call.

What fueled this obsession? Maybe it's the primal scream against the dying of the light. Or perhaps it's the love affair with life's every joy and sorrow, and the unwillingness to let it all slip away. We've grasped at alchemy and the Philosopher's Stone, at the fabled Fountain of Youth, and at the elixirs of Chinese emperors—all spiritual GPS coordinates for humanity's homing instinct toward eternity.

We haven't stopped; our modern world is just another chapter in this ongoing tale. We're probing the DNA helix like it's the language of the gods, whispering the secrets of aging. And "You are what you eat"? That was never just about nutrition—it's a mantra for the possibility that, if you play your biochemical cards right, you might just outlast the rat race of cells ticking toward their expiration date.

Go back to the times of the ancient Egyptians, and you see a civilization captivated by the afterlife. They wrapped their deceased in bandages, believing against belief that flesh could be made eternal. Step forward to the Greeks and find philosophers musing over the immortality of the soul, transcending the crude decay of the body.

It wasn't always about the individual, either. Sometimes, it was about legacy, about leaving a mark immortalized in the minds of those to come. The Romans built their roads straight and their monuments grand, convinced that bricks and marble could withstand the assault of time far better than flesh and blood.

Entering the Dark and Middle Ages, things get mystical. Monks hunched over ancient texts, whispering incantations, and crafting amulets that promised more than protection—they offered a sliver of hope for life extension. These were not merely trinkets; they were beacons of human defiance against the march of mortality.

And it's not just the folks in the timeline behind us; it's the visionaries sprinting forward. From Ponce de León setting sail to unknown lands on a hunch, to the science fiction writers who cast their minds out to the cosmos. They pitch us stories where cryonics and stasis fields suspend life in limbo until a future age can rekindle the spent torch of existence.

This thirst for immortality has been a siren call that, for all its romance, also has its edges dipped in dread and unease. Maybe that's because deep down, we suspect that nature guards the secret of eternal life like the most jealous of dragons—serene in the knowledge that the game is rigged in favor of entropy.

Yet, if history has taught us anything, it's that people won't stop trying. It's not so much about outrunning death as it is about catching up with life—in all its infinite complexities and passions. That's what we're really chasing when we reach for immortality: an endless dawn to fulfill the promises we make to ourselves under starlit skies, an infinity of tomorrows to love, to learn, and to simply be.

Chapter 2: The Science of Aging

Now, let's dive deep into the nuts and bolts of why we age because, honestly, it's a puzzle that's both fascinating and maddening, isn't it? Think about it: our bodies are these incredibly complex systems that tick along like well-oiled machines, yet as time ticks on, those same systems start to sputter and slow down. But why? That's what we need to wrap our heads around. On this winding road, we'll tackle the cellular culprits that make our skin wrinkle and our hair gray. It's a blend of genetic coding—kind of like a biological script handed down through generations—and the environmental jazz that plays out in various ways, depending on your life's soundtrack. Picture this: DNA replication is a bit like hitting the copy button over and over until the quality starts to degrade. Makes sense, right? Then there are the baddies, like oxidative stress—think of it as rust for your cells. But don't get discouraged; real progress is being made in the lab, breakthroughs that could one day turn the tables on Father Time. So while we may not have a fountain of youth just yet, who's to say that science won't one day provide a map to those elusive waters?

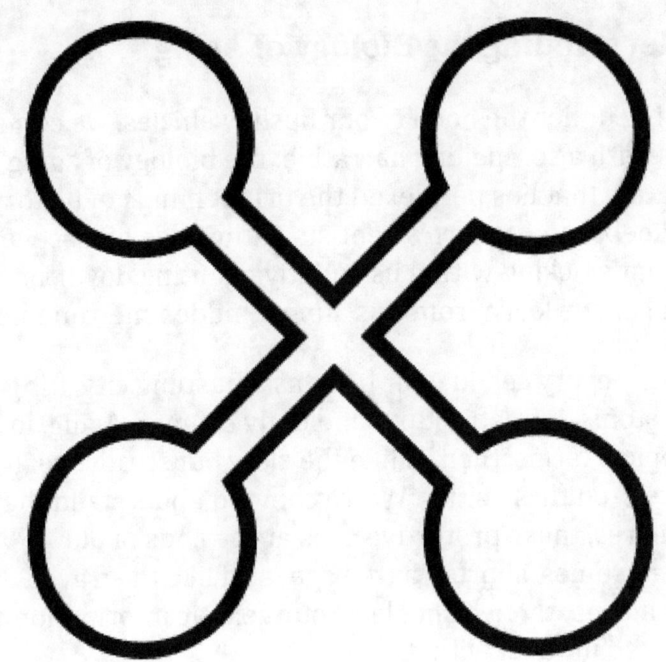

Understanding the Biology of Aging

Peering under the hood of our fleshy vehicles, we come to grips with a compelling narrative: the biology of aging. It's a tale that has perplexed the bright minds of history and keeps our modern scientists at the edge of discovery. So what's ticking within us, quietly counting down, and what can we learn from this almost hidden metronome?

Imagine every cell in your body as a bustling city, it's got its systems, infrastructure, and daily dramas. Aging, in biological terms, then, is like the slow but steady wear and tear on these cities. We've come to understand that telomeres, those protective caps at the ends of our chromosomes, shorten as we age. And like the frayed end of a once neatly tied shoelace, our genetic information begins to unravel with it.

It's not just about what's going wrong either; it's about what's not happening right anymore. Autophagy, a tidy-up process where our cells recycle and trash the junk, tends to get a bit lazy as we clock in more years. Picture the garbage collectors striking and you're seeing the cluttered streets of our cells as they age.

And who's not fascinated by the genetics of it all? You've got these longevity genes, sirtuins, and FOXOs acting as the body's own fountain of youth—if only we could tap into them more effectively. They're like those rare, mystical herbs in ancient tales, promising vigor and life, except they're real and coded snug within our DNA, waiting for science to whisper the secrets of their activation.

Then there's this theory, the mitochondrial clock of aging, which hints at a power struggle at the cellular level. Free radicals, those pesky molecular rebels, deal damage to our powerhouses, the mitochondria, leading to a cascade of energy deficits that ripple through our vitality. It's an internal battle that we are just starting to understand how to mediate.

But let's not ignore the external players in this drama. Oxidative stress and inflammation are like the relentless elements battering the external walls of our cellular cities. Over time, the relentless assault can break down even the strongest of defenses, leading to chronic diseases synonymous with the ticking clock of life.

We've also got glycation, a process where sugar molecules bulldoze their way into proteins and DNA, gumming up the works. It's like throwing sand into an engine; everything slows down, grinds, and eventually wears out. Reducing sugar intake may seem obvious in light of this, but the biological Dorian Gray within us will need more than just diet alterations to keep the portrait unblemished.

As we navigate these processes, we establish a map of aging, charting the decline like explorers in reverse, plotting a journey back from the weary elder to the wide-eyed youth. The hope is that by backtracking, we find the junctures where we can intervene, perhaps tweak a gene here, enhance an enzyme there, or lift the siege upon a mitochondrion to recover the lost territory of youth.

Are we rewriting the final chapters of life's book? Yes, and no. Intervening in the aging process feels less like a revision and more like understanding the original text in its ancient, whispering language. It's a code we're born with and carries within us the potential for extending the narrative of our lives in ways that still fit the natural order—just with a little more longevity as the side effect.

Understanding the biology of aging is foundational to the latter chapters of our exploration. It sets the stage for the breakthroughs in anti-aging research, the mind-body optimizations, and technological wizardry to come. By delving deep into our biological realities, we arm ourselves with knowledge—one that leads us through the rest of this saga where science edges closer to the once mythical realm of everlasting life.

Genetic and Environmental Factors that Contribute to Aging

Digging into the trenches of the aging process, it's like peeling back the layers of an infinite onion. You can't help but get teary-eyed at the complexity of it all. We're talking genes dancing with environment in a tango where each step counts – a delicate balance that ultimately leads down the path to aging. And what a profound journey it is. Understanding these factors isn't just about hitting the brakes on the aging process; it's about tuning the orchestra of our biology so that each note resonates with vitality.

Every cell in our body holds the genetic blueprint that can either be our ticket to longevity or the weak link in our armor. We inherit DNA from our parents – the good, the bad, and the unruly. Some of us get dealt a royal flush with genes that bless us with a sturdy heart and a brain that stays sharp as a tack well into our golden years. Others might carry genetic variants that whisper the promises of longevity, but like a secret that's only revealed with the right handshake, environmental factors need to play their part.

Our environment is a sprawling stage where our genes are either the stars of the show or the understudies waiting in the wings. The sun kissing your skin, that deep breath of mountain air, or the smog you inhale during rush hour traffic – they're all cues, nudges that can wake up those genetic potentials or tell them to hit the snooze button. Lifestyle choices are the directors in this play, with nutrition calling the shots on how your body repairs itself and exercise deciding how strong your heart stays amidst the toils of time.

Picture stress as the antagonist in this plot, the nemesis lurking in the shadows, ready to turn your genes against you. Chronic stress doesn't just mess with your vibe; it flips switches in your DNA that can lead to inflammation, heart disease, and a brain that's not as sharp as it used to be. It's like throwing a wrench in the intricate machinery of your cells, causing wear and tear in places you can't even see.

Now, imagine antioxidants as the cavalry, riding in with all their might from the food we eat. They duke it out with free radicals – those unruly molecules that are bent on causing chaos like a bunch of graffiti artists tagging your cells with damage. Antioxidants are like the neighborhood watch, keeping things clean and maintaining order.

Yet, while we have this dance of genes and lifestyle, there's more to this aging narrative. The environment isn't just about what's on your plate or how much you deadlift at the gym. It's also the zip code you're born into, the air quality around you, the noise levels, and the societal stresses that can either pave a runway for a smooth take-off or create hurdles that you've got to jump over every day.

One can't help but wonder, are we simply marionettes tied to the strings of our genetics and the stage of our environment? Here's the kicker: there's a plasticity to it all. A hope that maybe through the right interventions – a tweak here, a nudge there – we can tip the scales in our favor. Epigenetics tells us that our actions and experiences can tag our DNA with molecular Post-it notes, changing how our genes are expressed without altering the genetic code itself.

It's not about turning back the clock but rather ensuring that each tick is robust, unwavering, and filled with quality. To harness both our genetic predispositions and environmental interactions, is to play the long game towards extending the very essence of who we are. It's this harmonious synchrony between our genes and our surroundings that plays a monumental part in the orchestra of aging, each factor a note in the symphony that is our lifespan.

And just as we must tune our instruments and practice our scales, we must nurture our body and mind with the environment it interacts with – be it through the foods that fuel us, the air that fills our lungs, or the stress that tests our resilience. It's a balancing act of such finesse that requires awareness, intention, and perhaps a bit of grace.

So, as we uncover more about how genetic and environmental factors waltz together through our lifetime, it's certain that this dance isn't merely a predetermined routine. It's a performance open to improvisation, to moments of jazz where we can step in and influence the longevity of our own show. It's about understanding the rules of the game so profoundly that we make them work for us, ultimately extending our time under the limelight of existence, vibrant and alive.

Breakthroughs in Anti-Aging Research

Peel back the layers of history, filled with elixirs of life and fountains of youth, and we land smack in the middle of the 21st century, where science isn't just flirting with the idea of slowing aging—it's getting into a full-blown affair. Let's dive headfirst into the pool of recent breakthroughs that have had lab coats rustling with excitement. It's a brave new world, replete with innovative research that's reshaping what we thought we knew about getting old.

Picture this: microscopic janitors traveling through your bloodstream, cleaning up the cellular debris that accumulates with time. These aren't the characters of a sci-fi novel, they're senolytics—agents specifically designed to target and destroy senescent cells, the zombielike cells that refuse to die yet no longer function correctly. They're implicated in everything from wrinkles to arthritis to heart disease. Recent studies leveraging these senolytics have shown promising results, pushing us to question the boundaries of human health span.

But let's take a step back and ponder the idea of our telomeres—the protective tips of our chromosomes that shorten as we age, much like the burning wick of a candle. Enter the enzyme telomerase, the metaphorical snuffer that can extend the wick's life. Here's the kicker: some preliminary studies suggest we might be able to activate telomerase to elongate telomeres, potentially putting a pause on part of the aging process. It's a balancing act though, as over activation can teeter us into dangerous territory, like cancer. So it's a game of precision, one that researchers are learning to navigate.

Let's not forget the mavericks of longevity, sirtuins. These proteins are like the conductors of an orchestra, ensuring each part of the cell plays in harmony—a symphony of proper metabolism, DNA repair, and more. With molecules like resveratrol (yes, that's the one found in red wine), we're discovering ways to boost the activity of these sirtuins, nudging our cells towards a more 'youthful' state.

Now, in the realm of diet, intermittent fasting has parachuted its way into public consciousness. But what's the science behind it? It turns out that fasting regimes can kick start cellular autophagy—the body's way of cleaning out damaged cells to make way for new ones—like hitting the reset button on your body's cellular integrity. It's a hotbed of research with the potential to transform not just lifespans but the quality of those extra years.

And let's lace up our boots and march into the battlefield of the gut microbiome, host to trillions of bacteria that could hold sway over our longevity. Each trip to the fridge might as well be a diplomatic mission to this microcosmic civilization within us. Emerging studies are establishing links between gut health and age-related diseases, and paving the way for targeted probiotics that could restore gut flora to that of our sprightly younger selves.

Of course, there's the basilisk in the room—an entwined creature called genetics. CRISPR, the gene-editing wizardry that has taken the research world by storm, promises customized interventions in our genetic code that could knock out predispositions to age-related diseases or possibly introduce beneficial mutations that extend lifespan.

Amidst these breakthroughs, we're also tapping into the regenerative power of stem cells, coaxing them to repair and replace tissues that time has worn down. From Parkinson's to heart disease, from mending spinal cords to regrowing hair, stem cells stand as one of the heavyweight champions in the arena of anti-aging research.

Now hold on, what about the brain, the crown jewel of our being? Advances in neuroplasticity have uncovered that our brains aren't set in stone but are malleable, capable of growth and repair throughout our lives. Through cognitive training, lifestyle changes, and maybe even future interventions, we might preserve our mental acuity as the years tick by.

As we strap on our goggles and peer into the petri dish of immortality, these breakthroughs paint an exciting picture. We're not just on the verge of slowing aging; we're tinkering on the cusp of flipping it on its head. Lean in closely, because each day whispers new promises of youth preserved and life extended, and somewhere in that complex intersection of cells and science lies the tantalizing possibility of stretching the tape at the finish line of life itself.

Chapter 3: Mind and Body Optimization

Lingering on the edge of breakthroughs in anti-aging from the previous chat, we now dive head first into the yin and yang of longevity: mind and body optimization. Think of your brain as the maestro leading the orchestra of your bodily functions with the precision of a Swiss watch. It's in the daily grind, the nitty-gritty of our routines, that the magic happens. What if refining mental gymnastics and flexing your cerebral muscles could not just fend off age but give you a mental edge sharp enough to slice through the fog of years? And let's marry that to the temple that is your body, through the discerning art of exercise, the science of superfoods, and the ritualistic beauty of consistent, healthful lifestyle choices. This twin-engine approach isn't just about extending the timeline. It's about enhancing the quality of each tick, and tock, of that timeline, ushering in a symphony of life-quality that crescendos with each vibrant year passed. Here, we explore the tactics and habits that can fortify the fort of your body and polish the mirror of your mind, because in the pursuit of immortal vigor, it's not only about how long you live, but the richness with which you experience every moment of that life.

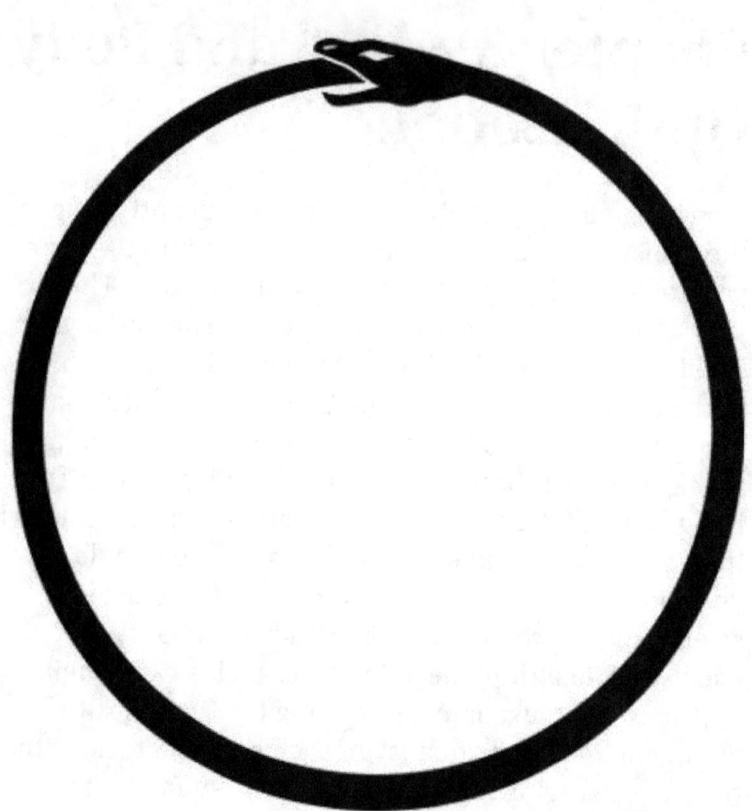

Mental and physical health as keys to longevity

The mind and body are deeply interconnected; a reality that's both ancient wisdom and cutting-edge science. On this journey towards unlocking the secrets of immortality, it's crucial to hone in on the yin-yang duo of mental and physical health. It's like nurturing the roots of a tree—the stronger they are, the higher and lusher it can grow.

Let's dive into the cerebral pool for a sec. Mental health isn't just a buzzword; it's the scaffolding that supports our entire being. Stress, anxiety, depression – these are not just emotional states. They're chemical reactions, and they have real, tangible effects on our body's biology. Chronic stress can be just as damaging as smoking a pack a day or surviving on a diet of fast food. Our brain's health dictates the release of hormones and neurotransmitters that regulate everything from our heart rate to our immune system.

Now flip the coin, and you've got your physical health staring you down, begging for attention. Regular exercise, a balanced diet, staying hydrated—they're not revolutionary concepts, but put them into practice, and they can be transformative. The body's well-being fuels the mind, and believe me, a well-oiled machine keeps the gears in your head spinning smoothly.

Consider this: when you're physically active, you're not just building muscle and burning calories. You're pumping out endorphins, boosting your mood, and stoking the fires of your brain cells. The heart beats with more gusto, sending oxygen-rich blood rocketing through your veins, and powering up those neural pathways.

Oh, and let's talk food – because let's be real, food is life. Nutrition isn't just about managing weight; it's about selecting the premium fuel for our complex biological machinery. Antioxidants, micronutrients, omega-3 fatty acids, these aren't just fancy terms to nod at – they are the janitors of your body, cleaning up the mess and reducing inflammation, the silent killer that creeps up on you and messes with your longevity game plan.

It's not just about living longer; it's about living stronger, brighter, with a fire that doesn't flicker out. It's about standing up to Father Time and saying, "I'm not just going to stick around; I'm going to thrive." That's where mental acuity and emotional resilience come into play. Cognitive exercises, meditation, mindfulness – they're the bicep curls for your brain, keeping it nimble and quick, well into the golden years.

But hey, don't just nod along and then forget everything you've read. Integrate these practices into your life. Make them habitual, your new status quo. Small, day-to-day choices add up; like compound interest, they build upon each other, and before you know it, you've amassed a wealth of health.

Remember, isolation is the enemy of improvement. Connection, community – these are essential for mental fortitude. Don't cocoon yourself off. Find your tribe, engage, laugh, challenge each other. The human element can't be overstated; we're social creatures, and our inter-personal connections deeply influence our mental, and consequently, physical health.

And amidst this quest to body-mind optimization, let's not ignore the rhythm of life. Rest and recovery are not just breaks; they're active components of health-building.

Sleep, that magical slice of each day, is where the body repairs, the mind consolidates memories, and hormones balance themselves out. Skimp on it, and soon enough, the cracks start to show.

So as you step forth from this page and continue on this exploration of longevity, keep the mental-physical health dynamic in the forefront. Treasure it, nurture it, challenge it – and watch as each passing year becomes less about the number and more about the vitality you carry within you.

Strategies for optimizing brain function and cognitive health

Diving deep into our inner workings, it's imperative we talk about fine-tuning that grand conductor of our bodily orchestra: the brain. Maximizing our cognitive prowess isn't just about being sharp today; it's about ensuring our mental gears are oiled well into the twilight of our days. But how do we keep the cogs turning smoothly, you ask? Well, it's a delicate dance of habits, choices, and a little bit of science-backed strategy. Let's explore.

First up, hitting the lights on the subject of sleep. Yeah, the thing we often skimp on when life gets hectic. Yet, proper sleep is not just a luxury; it's the brain's non-negotiable time to hit the reset button. Quality Z's are like a spa day for your neurons, washing away mental cobwebs and buffering against cognitive decline. So, tonight, maybe think twice before binge-watching another series, eh?

Food for thought—literally. Those leafy greens and vibrant berries aren't just Instagram-worthy; they're loaded with antioxidants, battling the brain's archenemies: oxidative stress and inflammation. Omega-3 fatty acids? Bring 'em on. Not just for your heart, these slick nutrients are your brain's building blocks for maintaining cell membrane integrity and fighting off the fog of aging. Eat with intention—your brain will thank you.

Now let's lace up and talk exercise. But don't worry; I'm not about to scream "no pain, no gain" at you. However, the link between breaking a mild sweat and boosting brainpower is undeniable. Cardio isn't just for your heart; it pumps oxygen-rich blood to that gray matter upstairs, nourishing it with each stride, providing a neuroprotective edge we can't ignore. So take that brisk walk, yeah? Your future self might just outwit your past.

Never underestimate the beef between stress and your cerebral circuits. Chronic stress is like a relentless squall, battering your brain's ability to regenerate and retain its plasticity. But here's the silver lining: practices like mindfulness and meditation aren't just New Age fluff. They're your front-line defense, diffusing stress's stranglehold and keeping your mind supple. A little introspection might just be your cerebral shield.

Don't let lifelong learning collect dust like an old yearbook. The brain craves novelty—new skills, languages, puzzles. Challenge it, and it repays you in kind with neurogenesis and a resilience that scoffs at the years piling on. Curiosity didn't kill the cat; it gave it nine lives, so to speak. So go on, pick up that guitar gathering dust, or that language app you thought you were too old for. Surprise yourself.

Social butterflies might just be on to something. No, not just for the gossip but for weaving a web of cognitive fortifications. Engagements, community, heartfelt chats— not only do they enrich life, but they are also our brain's exercise, reinforcing memory and empathy networks. Loneliness isn't just a hollow feeling; it's a risk factor, and those laughs with friends are more protective than you may realize.

Then there's the matter of the mind's elixirs, in moderation, of course—things like caffeine and certain nootropics. They're not miracle potions, but when used judiciously, they can give you that edge; a sharper focus, a quicker wit. But always with caution—we're playing a long game here, no need for quick fixes that could backfire. Understand what you're fueling your mind with; knowledge is power, after all.

We can't ignore the landscape of our minds; mental health is paramount. Anxiety, depression, the spectres that haunt the recesses—addressing them isn't weakness; it's fortification. Therapy, self-awareness, emotional intelligence—these are tools, not crutches. We need to destigmatize the quest for mental wellness; our cognitive longevity depends on it.

Finally, the promise of our digital age—brain-training apps, virtual reality cognitive exercises—they're not just games. They are the frontiers of mental fitness, tailored challenges that adapt to our growing capabilities. As in bodybuilding, we progressively overload, but with bits and bytes. It's a brave new world for mental gymnastics, and we are its athletes.

So there it is—the gist of neural optimization. It's a mix of old wisdom and new science, of sweat and serenity, of community and the quest within. The brain is the crown jewel in longevity's quest, and it demands respect, reverence, and, yes, a bit of indulgence in the pleasures of life. After all, a life endlessly prolonged without the spice of vivid thought wouldn't be much of a life, would it? It's about quality, vibrancy, and with every intention, a dance that outlasts the setting sun.

Exercise, nutrition, and lifestyle choices for extending lifespan

Now, let's dive into the brass tacks of prolonging our dance with time through exercise, nutrition, and those critical everyday choices. If we ponder the idea that our bodies are the most sophisticated pieces of machinery we'll ever own, then it's a no-brainer that what we feed it and how we treat it will drastically affect its performance and longevity. It's not about fad diets or relentless gym routines; it's about sustainable, mindful choices that fuel our journey towards longevity.

Exercise isn't merely a tool for weight management—think of it as the ultimate tune-up for your biological engine. Regular physical activity has been linked to a decrease in all-cause mortality. But don't think you have to become an ultra-marathoner here. Consistency beats intensity when it comes to increasing your lifespan. It's about the sweet spot—integrating both aerobic and strength training exercises into a regular, manageable routine that keeps your heart, muscles, and joints in peak condition without burning out.

When it comes to eating, visualizing your diet as the premium gas you're selecting for your high-performance vehicle isn't too far off the mark. But there's no one-size-fits-all here; you've got to listen to your body's signals. Nutrient-dense foods, those packed with vitamins, minerals, and antioxidants, combat inflammation, which is essentially the body's version of rust. Colorful vegetables, lean proteins, healthful fats, and whole grains—they're the all-stars when fueling our internal powerhouse for longer life.

But, you might ask, what about when life gets chaotic? Stress management isn't just a trendy topic on mindfulness blogs; it's a cornerstone of longevity. Chronic stress is like sand in your engine—it's gritty, abrasive, and will wear down parts if not managed properly. Techniques ranging from mindfulness meditation to simply taking a walk in nature can dial down the body's stress response and give our cellular repair mechanisms a fighting chance to work their rejuvenating magic.

And hey, don't underestimate the impact of sleep. Skimping on shut-eye is like skipping oil changes; you wouldn't do that to a car you want to keep humming into the future, right? A solid seven to nine hours a night is part of that perfect maintenance regimen, sweeping away the brain's metabolic debris and repairing cellular damages endured throughout the day.

Lifestyle factors, such as alcohol consumption and smoking, absolutely affect the longevity equation. Picture pouring sugar into your gas tank; that's what smoking does over the long haul. As for alcohol, a splash of moderation can potentially be beneficial, but overindulgence? That's corrosive over time.

Never overlook the power of social connections and a sense of community. Just as a car would rust out sitting unused in a garage, isolation and loneliness can corrode the human spirit. Cultivating and maintaining relationships isn't just food for the soul; it literally influences biological processes, including inflammation and blood pressure, which impact longevity.

Then there's the sun—the great giver of life, but also a force that can damage if we're not cautious. Moderate sun exposure boosts vitamin D, but too much sun is like skipping the coolant and running the engine too hot; damage occurs over time, both visible and molecular.

Lastly, never forget that our bodies are continuously regenerating, with a resilience that needs pushing and testing to be sustained. Jump into cold water, get a little dirty in the garden, challenge your body and mind in new ways. It's a touch of the fight-or-flight without overdoing it—an occasional stressor that keeps the body's repair systems agile and responsive.

It's this interconnected web of actions and choices that threads through the fabric of our existence, where the physical meets the mental, the food meets the cells, and the social meets the biological. Endeavor to balance, to listen, to adjust, and to fine-tune your way toward a richer, fuller, longer life. The crossroads of all these paths may just lead us closer to the fountain of youth we've been seeking since time immemorial.

Chapter 4: Technological Advancements

Imagine diving into the deep end of a pool where the water isn't just water, but a fluid of endless innovation—this is what diving into the realm of technological advancements in anti-aging feels like. These days, it's not just about slapping on some anti-wrinkle cream and calling it a day; we're talking cutting-edge stuff that feels like it's straight out of a sci-fi novel. We've got scientists tinkering with our genetic codes like master locksmiths, hoping to find that sweet spot where aging gives up and keels over. Throw in some regenerative medicine—think growing new organs in a lab like you're baking a cake—and you can see why there's a tingling sense of excitement buzzing in the air. And don't even get me started on artificial intelligence; it's like the smart kid in class who's about to blow the curve for everybody, taking longevity research to places we've barely begun to fathom. It's a whirlwind of possibilities, each more mind-bending than the last, all converging to paint a picture of a future where 'forever young' isn't just a pipe dream—it's on the to-do list.

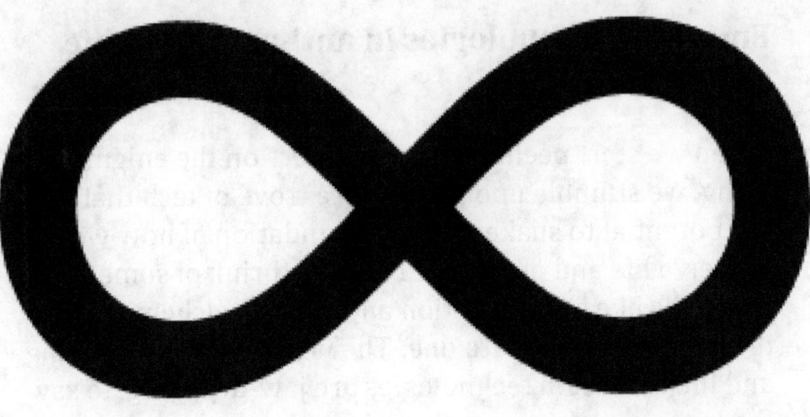

Emerging technologies in anti-aging and life extension

When we start peeling back the layers on the enigma of aging, we stumble upon a treasure trove of tech that's got the potential to shake the very foundation of how we perceive life and death. We're on the brink of something that feels like science fiction and ancient alchemical dreams all mashed into one: The next wave of anti-aging and life extension technologies are jaw-dropping, to say the least.

Picture this: tiny nanobots coursing through your bloodstream, repairing cells, zapping diseases, and basically, doing a tune-up on the fly. That's not some pipe dream; it's nanotechnology, and it's one of the emerging arenas where the marriage of tech and medicine might grant us some extra trips around the sun. While it's still early days, the research is picking up pace, and the possibilities are branching out like the roots of an age-old tree.

Then, let's chat about CRISPR, shall we? It's like genetic word processing, snipping and editing DNA – the code of life – with a precision that's never been possible before. Tinkering at this level opens up whole avenues for the potential not just to prevent, but to reverse the signs of aging at their source. It's not all about looking good; it's about redefining the boundaries of human health span. Do we dare to dream of a day when our cells could be programmed to overcome the very notion of biological aging?

Stem cells are also the rising stars on the life extension stage. They've got this uncanny ability to become just about any cell you need, patching up the worn-out bits, encouraging the body to heal itself. Regenerative medicine, though no silver bullet, is steadily carving out its niche as an anti-aging heavyweight.

While we're at it, let's not forget the digital realm's love affair with anti-aging – artificial intelligence is turning heads in the longevity space. With deep learning, AI can spot patterns, predict outcomes, personalize medicine, and ultimately, could become our secret weapon in staying several steps ahead of the ticking clock.

But wait, there's more. Bioprinting organs, right? Imagine printers, but instead of spitting out pages, they're laying down layers of cells to build brand-new, personalized organs. Transplant lists could be a thing of the past if we can just print what we need on demand. Life extension doesn't get much more tangible than giving someone a fresh heart or liver when they need it the most.

Moving from the physical to the digital, there's this buzz about digital twins – creating a virtual copy of yourself that can be tested against drugs and treatments, predicting your unique body's reactions without you having to pop a single pill. It's like a rehearsal for your health, and it's fascinating to think where that might lead us.

Okay, feel the pulse of this conversation – it's racing, right? Anti-aging is moving faster than ever, spurred on by quantum computing's colossal capacity to crunch data, creating simulations and models that outrace even the most future-forward thinker's wildest dreams. This tech could be the game-changer, where 'what if' scenarios become 'why not' solutions.

Then there's the hard reality: technology isn't just shaping the future; it's rewriting the very code of life, weaving itself into our biology in ways that challenge what it means to be human. It begs us to ask, if we can extend life, how far will we push it? What does it mean for our souls if our bodies refuse to follow the once-immutable path towards decay?

And, as much as technology promises a fountain of youth, we're still grappling with the profound implications of these advancements. The dance between innovation and ethics is complex and, at times, unsettling. As we push the boundaries, as we edge ever closer to life extension realms once relegated to the realm of gods, we must brace ourselves for the beautiful and bizarre symphony of progress and its consequences.

In closing this slice on emerging technologies, we're reminded that every sunrise holds the promise of a new discovery that could unlock another secret to longevity. The quest for eternal life is as old as humanity itself, but today, it's awash with technology that's rewriting our final chapter with the tantalizing possibility of a sequel. Yet, as we stand on the precipice of potential immortality, let's not forget the essence of what it means to live – not just in terms of years, but in the depth and breadth of our experiences.

The potential of genetic engineering and regenerative medicine

Imagine we're walking through a gallery of the future; genetic engineering and regenerative medicine are the masterpieces showcasing our boundless potential. It's as if we've been handed the keys to our biological blueprint, sparking a revolution in how we approach our health and ultimately, our mortality. What we're seeing is not just incremental progress, these fields are catapulting us into realms of healing and enhancement we once deemed science fiction.

Genetic engineering is a bit like having the ultimate software update at our disposal. We're beginning to tweak genes with the precision of a master craftsman, addressing the very code that can make us prone to aging and disease. The use of CRISPR and gene therapy allows us to imagine a day when we can flip the switches of our genetic makeup to resist diseases that have plagued humanity for eons. And it's not just about prevention; we're talking about fixing what's broken. Picture a world where gene editing could reverse the damage of a genetic heart condition or halt the progression of neurodegenerative diseases in their tracks.

Then there's regenerative medicine. Think of it as the art of biological resurrection, enticing cells to renew themselves and restoring tissues and organs that have failed us. The implications are staggeringly beautiful. Stem cells, for example, serve as the body's repairmen, rebuilding and rejuvenating like nature's own nano-tech. Injecting these cells into damaged hearts, brains, or joints isn't just repairing wear and tear; it's part of a larger narrative where we're not just extending life but enhancing its quality.

It's all about the synergy, isn't it? Genetic engineering makes way for more potent and precise medical interventions, while regenerative medicine rebuilds and rejuvenates our worn-down parts. It's like we're hitting the refresh button at the cellular level, unveiling the possibility of new organs grown from our own cells—a personal factory of sorts for body parts without the risk of rejection. Imagine the liberation, the potential easing of organ shortages, the lives extended, and the sufferings alleviated.

There's a philosophical edge to wielding such power. We're not just tinkering with machinery; we're reshaping existence, dialing down the entropic clock of our cells. As we venture further, questions bubble up like a spring of profound curiosity. What does it mean for humankind if we hold the sculptor's chisel over the marble of our genes and tissues? How do we shape ourselves without losing the essence of what it means to be human?

But we have to be straight with ourselves; the road ahead isn't devoid of potholes. Issues like accessibility, ethical quandaries over design babies, and the socioeconomic rifts that such tech could widen—these are the hurdles we must clear thoughtfully. It's vital we navigate this with as much wisdom as technical prowess, maintaining a balance between progress and the values we hold dear.

Then there's the elephant in the room: our deep-rooted fear of playing god or nature, depending on one's spiritual or secular compass. However, if history has taught us anything, it's that humanity rarely shies away from the power to transform its environment, or itself. We're taking the reins on evolution and in doing so, we must tread lightly, embrace humility, and respect the profound responsibility that comes with such power.

As we speculate on the future, visions of engineered superhumans and eternal youth flood the imagination—it's enticing, exhilarating, and to be frank, a bit unnerving. We're on the cusp of rewriting the tale of human existence, nudging it ever closer to the once-unattainable desire for longevity and perhaps, immortality. What becomes crucial is ensuring that such profound advancements work not just for the privileged few, but for the betterment of all humanity, knitting a tapestry of life that is richer and fuller for everyone.

In wrapping up this glimpse into the future, let's circle back to the essence of it all—the very heartbeat of why we're drawn to extend our lives. It's not merely about more years on the clock, but about the experiences, the connections, the joys and sorrows, learning and loving. It's about the boundless curiosity that drives us to explore, grow, and indeed, to live. With genetic engineering and regenerative medicine, we're opening doorways to a future where our lifespan could reflect the enormity of our human spirit.

So, as we explore the myriad paths technology may lead us down, let's pivot with care but also with courage. Amidst the turbulence of such seismic shifts, it's the human touch, the shared stories, and the collective dream of a healthier, more vibrant life that must guide our way forward. Onward we go, into the rich unknown.

Artificial intelligence and its impact on longevity research

Let's dive in. The intersection of artificial intelligence and longevity research isn't just intriguing—it's potentially revolutionary. We're talking about a realm where cutting-edge algorithms meet the cellular secrets of aging. Imagine a world where AI can predict how changes in your DNA might play out over decades or can tailor a cocktail of interventions designed to slow the hands of time, just for you.

Today's longevity scientists aren't just toiling away in labs with test tubes and microscopes. They're partnering with AI—this silent, tireless, and incredibly smart collaborator. It's like having Sherlock Holmes on the case, but instead of solving crimes, it's deciphering the complex mysteries behind why we age and how we can stall it. AI algorithms digest massive datasets, see patterns we can't, and suggest hypotheses at a scale and speed that leave human capabilities in the dust.

So, this is the kind of partnership with a turbo boost. For example, AI can analyze genetic information from populations with unusual longevity, transpose it into actionable data, and then—bam—we can apply this to interventions. From genomic sequencing to the analysis of the metabolome, AI helps us identify longevity pathways that might have taken eons to uncover through human trial and error alone.

But it's not just about crunching numbers; AI is our creative partner, too. It generates models that can simulate complex biological processes, predict outcomes of potential therapies, and even design new molecules that could become the next big anti-aging drugs. It's like having a master builder who can see the blueprint of life and then tweak it, enhancing longevity piece by piece.

Consider the research on senescent cells—those pesky cellular squatters that accumulate with age and wreak havoc on your body. AI is helping us to map out these cellular Badlands, understand their effects, and develop senolytic drugs to clear them out. It's as if we're reprogramming the body's cleanup crew to be much more efficient, and AI is the foreman guiding the operation.

Longevity research with AI at the helm also means personalized medicine taken to the next level. No more one-size-fits-all; AI can factor in your unique genetic makeup, lifestyle, and even your gut microbiome to devise a longevity plan as distinctive as your fingerprint. It's like your personal health tailor, stitching together a perfect-fit solution for aging.

But wait, you might say, is it all rosy? Certainly not. There's the risk of data breaches, ethical quagmires, and misaligned AI models, which could lead to skewed interpretations. Vigilance and ethical frameworks aren't just wise; they're prerequisites to keep this powerful tool in line with our human values.

So, what about tomorrow? We're teetering on the brink of what could be the biggest breakthroughs in the history of longevity science, powered by AI. The AI of tomorrow could be designing complex, multi-drug regimens, continually optimizing them through real-time feedback loops from your body's sensors. Imagine a life where AI is your personal longevity coach, nudging you towards the optimal path for a healthy lifespan, not just in the clinic but daily, moment by moment.

It's no longer the stuff of science fiction; we're weaving the fabric of this future as we speak, each technological advancement a new thread in the tapestry of enhanced life. And as we explore this brave new world, we must keep the dialogue open, ethics tight and eyes on the prize—a world where aging is not a decline but a new beginning, rich with possibilities, guided by the wisdom of artificial intelligence.

The integration of AI into longevity research isn't just a leap forward; it's a visionary dance between human desire and machine intelligence. It's a partnership that asks us to be as brave and creative as the tools we wield, to sculpt a future where longevity is crafted with precision, care, and an understanding of life's immeasurable value.

Chapter 5: Ethical and Philosophical Considerations

Imagine you're having the time of your life, forever. Tempting, isn't it? But let's not get too carried away and forget to ponder the big picture. Ethics and philosophy, they're not just for academia's ivory towers; these are real, meaty chunks of thought we've got to chew on. Think of us grappling with the dicey idea of outliving our planet's resources, or the social quagmires of who gets to sip from the fountain of youth. Would you still crave immortality if only a chosen few could afford it? Philosophically, it's a minefield. Can we still be 'us' minus the visceral fear of death? If mortality's the mother of invention, what happens when we show her the door? Life's fabric is complex, woven with threads of moral conundrums and existential queries that deserve more than a skim. So, let's dive deep, contemplate the reality of a never-ending story, and its ramifications on how we love, learn, and let go.

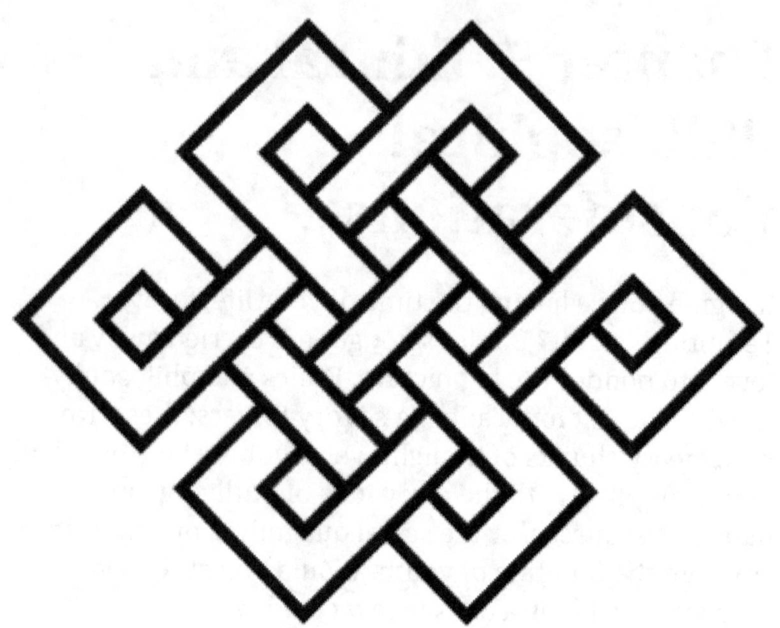

The implications of extended lifespans on society and the individual

Imagine, just for a second, what it would actually feel like to hit triple digits... and beyond. It's not just about blowing out a sea of candles on your birthday cake every year, but grappling with everything that extra time does to your mind, your relationships, your society. Extended lifespans aren't just a cool possibility; they're a game-changer that digs deep into the fabric of our existence.

So, what happens when we start racking up years like never before? Well, for starters, the whole dynamic of 'getting older' gets a major facelift. If you're the kind that gnaws on existential questions, picture how the extra time'll reshape your bucket list. That 'carpe diem' vibe might mellow down 'cause, hey, you've got centuries to hit those goals, right? But then, think about the flip side; will ambition fade when the tick-tock of the biological clock isn't as loud?

Let's take a second and talk society—it's not just chilling in the backseat here. Imagine the workforce...alive and kicking, well past the current retirement age. It's a double-edged sword. Experience stays on the payrolls longer, but does it jam the upward mobility for the young guns? And with people having more time, will they pivot careers like they're swapping out clothes? Emergent studies might be needed just to keep this longevity train chugging smoothly on the tracks of an evolving job market.

Then there are relationships—till death do us part might need a new clause for the millennium-long marriage. Think about it. What does love look like when 'forever' could be, quite literally, forever? Not to mention friendships; they could ebb and flow in ways we can't even wrap our heads around yet. Lifetime bonds might be just the first act in a marathon rien ne presse drama.

Have you considered the fabric of family? Already complex, its weave could become unfathomable. Generations would overlap in unprecedented ways, and ancestry could become akin to a living library rather than just a family tree. Those ties that bind might be stretched to new lengths as families expand across extended timescales.

And what about the global stage? Longer lifespans could tweak the play of geopolitics like it's nobody's business. Leaders with more time to affect change—or chaos—and populations that swell without end could make for an international telenovela too tangled for simple solutions. World resources? Brace yourself; we're in for a bumpy ride unless innovation can match the voracious appetite of a growing, aging, ever-thirsty populace.

Let's not forget personal identity either. It undergoes evolution with the mere passage of a few years. But expand that to a century or more? The person you are at 25 versus 225 might look like day and night. It's not just your wardrobe that's gonna need an overhaul. Philosophies, beliefs, personal narratives—they're all in for a long, strange trip. The quest for purpose could become less a sprint, and more like those endless desert highways that make you wonder if the horizon will ever show up.

And just for a moment, entertain the thought of social order. With the gift of time, might there emerge a new hierarchy based not on wealth or status, but on age and wisdom? Yet, in the same breath, we've got to wrestle with whether prolonged life will steepen already sky-high disparities. Will immortality be the ultimate VIP pass, or could it be the wildcard to level the playing field once and for all?

Nudging the philosophical envelope a bit further, consider the soul's journey. If we're clocking in centuries, does that alter fundamental spiritual beliefs and practices? Do we start to view our stints on Planet Earth differently when the exit isn't just around the corner? It's not just religious traditions that might need a revamp; the very ethos of life carries the potential for a seismic shift.

So, take a deep breath and let it all marinate. We're staring down a future that might just dangle the carrot of eternity in front of us. Buckling down for a couple of decades is one thing, but navigating the labyrinth of consequences that come with stretching our stay here? That's a whole other odyssey. And here we are, just dipping our toes into what could truly be the waters of forever.

Ethical dilemmas surrounding immortality and life extension

Imagine we've cracked the code, sipped from the modern-day Fountain of Youth, and bang, we've got a shot at immortality or at least a drastically expanded lifespan. This isn't your typical sci-fi flick—this is the real potential future, mixed with a side of ethical brain benders that need some serious chewing over.

So, let's start with the hot potato, inequality. Extend life for a few, and suddenly you've got an immortal elite class lapping up centuries of life like it's a bottomless mimosa brunch. These lucky folks might stack up wealth, influence, and know-how, leaving the rest in the dust with their measly eighty-odd years. It paints a stark picture when you imagine society fractured along lines forged by access to life-extending tech.

Then there's the question of overpopulation. A planet already creaking under the weight of seven billion souls gets no relief if nobody's making an exit. Space and resources are finite, my friend, and we need to wrestle with what it means to keep adding chairs to Earth's dinner table without ever saying goodbye to a single guest. It's like organizing a party and everyone RSVPs 'yes' without an end time. The cupcakes won't last, will they?

What about Mother Nature's tried and tested playbook: evolution? If aging takes a back seat, our genetic exchange becomes a sluggish affair. We might be staring down the barrel of stunted biological progress, snoozing our way through an evolutionary standstill. Natural selection has been the driving force behind our survival and adaptability, but eternal life could slam the brakes on this wild ride.

But wait, there's a human angle we can't ignore. Love, loss, and legacy. With longer lifelines, we'd witness an emotional conundrum unfold. Relationships stretch over centuries, and the pain of losing someone could become a rare beast, twisting the very fabric of how we experience grief and attachment. Plus, how do you shape a legacy if you're just going to stick around? The concept of leaving something behind loses its luster when you're in no hurry to depart from the party.

What's more, there's dignity in the natural arc of life. Each phase—youth, maturity, old age—holds value and lessons. If we're forever young or perpetually middle-aged, you have to wonder what we lose from the cycle. Those golden years, the time when reflection and wisdom bloom, might become extinct, reducing human existence to an endless loop where the focus is always on what's next rather than what has been.

Okay, and we can't sidestep the big one: meaning. Many of us claw through life driven by the tick-tock of that mortal clock. It's the urgency that gets us up in the morning, lights our entrepreneurial fires, and has us scratching down bucket lists. Strip away the deadline, and do we risk a diluted existence where tomorrow is always another day, and aspirations drift into procrastination?

Virtues, too, can take a hit. Patience, perseverance, and resilience—qualities honed by life's fleeting nature—are in jeopardy if we live through centuries of sunrises. It's possible we become less human, having ejected the heart-thumping awareness that time is precious.

And let's not forget responsibility. We're already not the greatest at tending to our yard when it comes to the environmental mess we're making; would immortality make us better stewards or would it embolden our reckless streak? Will someone living for hundreds of years look at climate change as their issue to solve, or would they think, "Eh, it'll sort itself out eventually"?

Navigating the legal minefield that comes with agelessness is another fun one. Laws, retirement, inheritance—society's infrastructure would need one heck of a renovation if death stops knocking. It's not just about slapping on a fresh coat of paint; it's a total overhaul of the systems that have kept societal gears grinding for eons.

So, this dream of living to see countless tomorrows is twisted up with threads of moral, social, and philosophical knots. It's a wild mix of potential and problem, a tapestry we must weave with care to avoid unraveling the essence of what it means to be human. Every step towards that immortal horizon has to be measured, every advancement bearing the weight of consequence. After all, forever is only worth it if it's worth living well, for all, with wisdom at the wheel and humanity at heart.

Philosophical perspectives on the nature of life and death

Ever thought about life and death? I mean, really chewed on it, rolled it around in your mind like a piece of hard candy, getting down to the nitty-gritty of what it all means? Well, let's take a deep dive into the philosophical rabbit hole where the ideas about life's essence and death's inevitability have been marinated in human thought for, like, forever.

The big question that's kept philosophers up at night is whether life is essentially something more than the sum of its parts. We're biological beings, sure, but is there a sprinkle—no, a downpour—of something extra, something intrinsic that keeps the gears turning? The nature of life has been described in countless ways: as a journey, a battle, a dance, a gift. And that's just scratching the surface. Each perspective helps us understand the layers and textures of our existence while highlighting the profound mystery at the core of living.

And when it comes to death, oh man, that's life's ultimate frenemy. Since the dawn of time, humans have wrestled with mortality's heavy cloak, trying to make peace with the daunting silence of non-existence. Is death the final curtain or simply an intermission? It has been depicted as a grim reaper, a welcome release, an eternal rest, the start of a different adventure in the afterlife, or an incomprehensible void. Pretty wild to think about, huh?

Now, imagine if we just hit pause on the whole process. The concept of life extension shakes the philosophical tree by asking what it means to stretch our time on this rock to the max. People have dreamed about immortality, jotting it down in myths and legends, perpetually tantalizing with its cocktail of hope and hubris. Life extension has us reevaluating the value of each moment when time becomes a potentially limitless commodity. Are we diluting the flavor of life experiences when we draw them out like taffy?

Let's take it a step further—such a radical shift in our lifespans sends a shockwave through our conventional wisdom on life's purpose. If life's a canvas and death's the frame that gives it meaning, what happens when that frame stretches out into eternity? Are we left with a droopy, saggy canvas, or do we find the beauty in creating art that never quite says 'The End'?

We've always been in this mad love affair with the concept of life meaning something profound. Is it about accumulating wisdom, enjoying a buffet of experiences, fulfilling a moral blueprint, or simply existing gracefully in the cosmos? Now add infinite time to the mix. Does life start to mean more, or does it kind of lose its edge? Philosophers from Socrates to Sartre have grappled with this, and still, we've got more soul-searching to do.

Oh, and let's not forget about the big D—death itself. What's up with that? Isn't there something to be said about its power to wrap up our existence with a neat (or not so neat) bow, giving the narrative arc of our intertwining tales a definite conclusion? It's been playing the role of the inevitable finales that shape our choices, our fears, our dreams. But, with our ever-improving tools and an unquenchable thirst for days that roll into more days, death's dominion might be up for grabs. Does that force us to rewrite the philosophical playbook on what it means to truly live and genuinely die?

Here's a curveball for you: eternity gets a bit gnarly when thinking about our identity. What parts of ourselves are intertwined with the dance of time? Our memories, our relationships, our ever-evolving selves—are they getting stretched thin, or are they expanding into a richer version? Identity over an infinite lifespan begs the question... are we still us, or something else entirely?

Shackled by the great unknown, we're left pondering about consciousness, the self, and continuity. If we crack the code to eternal life, does our consciousness continue to flow seamlessly, or does it evolve into something unrecognizable? Does the essence of who we are become a ghost in the shell of our potentially immortal bodies?

So, think about it—life, death, and the musings in between. Tear into it like a barbell session for your brain or a green smoothie for your soul. We're all about digging deep into these themes, not just to stir the pot but to simmer a stew of understanding that's seasoned with questions that might just define the trajectory of our species. And hey, when we're talking about the potential for endless tomorrows, who isn't intrigued by the possibilities?

Chapter 6: Practical Strategies for Longevity

Imagine this—you've been on a riveting journey through the labyrinth of immortality, twisted through the DNA helixes in search of the fountain of youth, and have now stumbled upon the treasure trove that is Chapter 6. In this chapter, we're grounding ourselves in the day-to-day grind, turning our gaze to the habits, the mindset, and the camaraderie that fortify the bridge to our aspirational longevity. You're going to find that it's the little things, the habitual sips of water, the mindful munching on a rainbow of veggies, and those deep, diaphragmatic breaths that potentially add years to the life odometer. And let's not sidestep the profound powers of laughter and connection; that balm for the soul that stitches the tapestry of a robust life narrative. Building a support network isn't just about having shoulders to lean on; it's about syncing heartbeats, sharing belly laughs, and forging the emotional resilience that shapes ironclad spirits. It's about waking up each day with anticipation for the subtle shifts toward a fuller, healthier existence. In this dance with time, each step, each groove is intentional, contributing to an ageless rhythm that echoes—every day is another chance to get it right, to oil the gears of longevity with practical, soulful living.

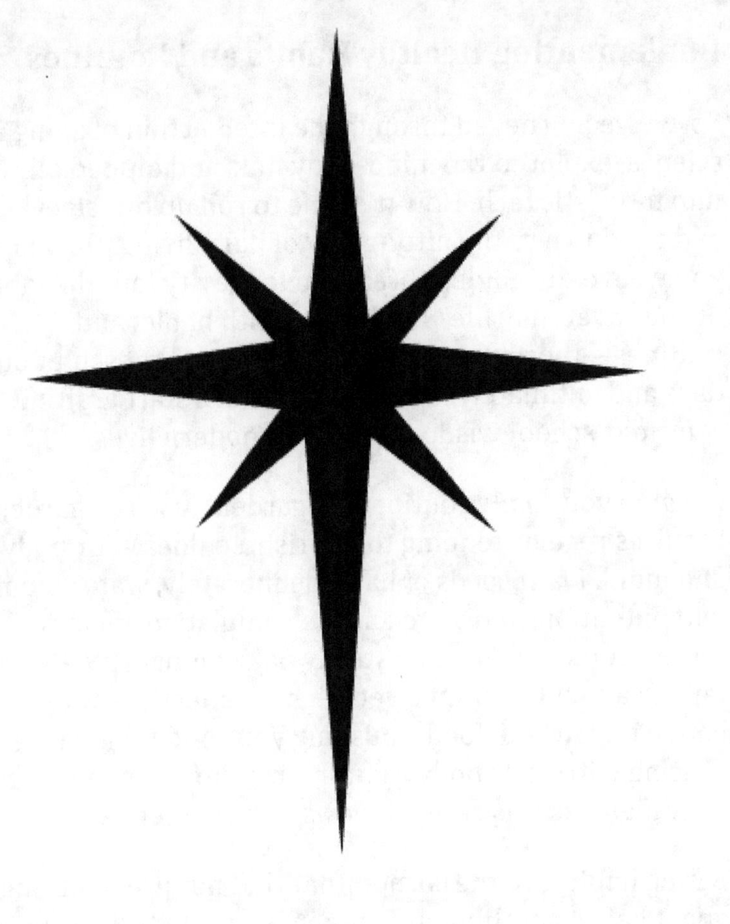

Implementing Healthy Habits and Routines

So, we've journeyed through the intersection of aging and science, explored the mind-body link, and dipped our toes into futuristic tech. Now it's time to roll up our sleeves and get down to the nitty-gritty of daily living. How do you weave the golden threads of longevity into the fabric of your everyday life? It all starts with habits and routines—those small, repetitive actions that sculpt our days and, ultimately, our lifespans. Let's start grafting some old-school wisdom onto our modern lives.

Imagine your daily routine as a garden. Just as a garden requires regular tending to flourish, so does your body and mind. Plant seeds of habit deliberately, water them with intention, and watch as the cumulative effect of these habits grows into a sturdy oak of longevity. We're talking about the simple yet mightily effective stuff— eating real, whole foods, pushing your body regularly, syncing with your body's natural rhythms, and ensuring your nights are as restorative as nature intended.

Eating habits are the cornerstone. I'm not just spouting about kale smoothies and quinoa bowls; let's focus on a variety of nutrient-dense foods that feel like a treat, not a chore. Think colorful veggies, lean proteins, a rainbow of fruits, healthy fats, and hydrating sips. Now, mix that up with intermittent fasting or time-restricted eating. There's a kind of magic in giving your digestive system a break, letting those cells focus on repair and rejuvenation instead of constantly churning through your latest snack.

Moving your body is just as crucial. It's not just about hitting the gym or clocking miles. We're looking for that sweet spot where exercise slots into life like your favorite playlist. Maybe it's dancing in your living room, hiking trails with friends, or sun salutations as the dawn creeps in. The high is real, my friends—the rush of endorphins, the surge of growth hormone. It's nature's elixir, and it's potent.

Ever consider your relationship with the sun and the moon? Our bodies are hardwired to rise with the sun and wind down as it sets. So, catch those morning rays for a dose of Vitamin D and to set that internal clock. At night, dim the lights, power down the screens, and let the moonlight signal your body to release melatonin, guiding you toward a deep sleep that's nothing short of a nightly renovation for your body.

Speaking of sleep, let's not forget the power of a peaceful slumber. Prioritizing sleep isn't laziness; it's one of the most robust longevity strategies known to humankind. Deep sleep is like pressing the reset button, scrubbing your brain clean of the day's toxins, and knitting your muscles and tissues back together. Develop a nightly ritual that quiets the mind and soothes the soul—a warm bath, a cup of herbal tea, or maybe just a good book and the sound of silence.

Mental fitness is just as pivotal. Call it what you will—meditation, mindfulness, contemplation—they're paths to the same destination. A clear, focused, and stress-hardy mind is a foundation you can't afford to overlook. Carve out a nook in your day for stillness. Breathe deeply, observe your thoughts without judgment, and center yourself. This isn't about escaping life; it's about plunging deeper into it, fully present and with a sense of tranquility that borders on the divine.

Your social garden needs tending too. Nurture relationships that sustain you. Connect with those who lift you up and support your goals—the ones who cheer you on when you're two bites into a kale salad and struggling to find the joy. Longevity isn't a lonesome road; it's a communal feast. Fill your table with love, laughter, and the kind of support that can't be measured, only felt.

Finally, let's not forget the power of setting intentions. Each morning is a new canvas—what will you paint today? Will it be a day structured around health, movement, and connection? Or will it be lost to the chaos of no plan? Set goals, however grand or modest, and let them guide your choices. Maybe it's as simple as drinking a little more water or as daring as trying a new fitness class. Whatever it is, let those aspirations be the compass that nudifies your path toward longevity.

In all, the art of establishing healthy habits and routines is a canvas constantly being painted. The brushes you use, the strokes you make, the colors you choose—they matter. Every healthy meal, every burst of exercise, every good night's sleep adds up. It stacks and layers into a mosaic of longevity—a life lived richly, purposefully, and perhaps, just perhaps, infinitely.

Mental and Emotional Practices for Promoting Longevity

Let's dive into the cerebral soup that's as crucial for longevity as any superfood or squat thrust. It's true, isn't it? The contentment in our heads and hearts can't be overlooked when we're chasing those extra candles on our birthday cake. Imagine the brain as a muscle, flexing with the heavy lifting of stress management, positive thinking, and deep connections.

It's like this—wielding mindfulness and emotional intelligence not only untangles the mental knots but also color-codes them for easier handling. Ever heard of neuroplasticity? That's the brain's crafty ability to adapt and rewire itself. Pressing pause on the harried pace of life to meditate isn't just navel-gazing; it shapes our brains to fend off the rust of aging. Peering inward, we sculpt neuronal pathways, boost mental resilience, and bathe in a soothing cocktail of brain-bolstering chemicals.

Consider the tapestry of our thoughts, woven with threads of optimism. A sunny disposition is more than a disposition; it's a buffer against the stormy weathers of life. Pessimism ages us like bread left out of the breadbox—stale and uninviting. So we kindle the flame of hope and laugh more; hey, it's like an internal jog for our organs, and a bright perspective keeps our cellular machinery humming longer and stronger.

But wait, it's not just about the solo journey. The heartbeat of our emotional wellness is connection. Loneliness isn't just a holler in the void; it's inflammatory, a slow-burn fire charring our longevity stakes. Build a tribe, foster relationships, and lean into the heart-to-hearts. Our social web is the safety net catching us when the high wire of life wobbles beneath our feet.

Let's talk stress, the sneaky thief of time robbing us of our youthful verve. Managing stress isn't about dodging life's curveballs—it's about cushioning the blow and bouncing back. It's empowering to realize that resilience is our internal Phoenix, rising from the ashes of our burnt-out selves. Techniques abound, from controlled breathing to coloring our worlds with hobbies that anchor us in tranquility.

Here's something else—ever noticed how empathy can be like a warm bath for the soul? Flexing our empathy muscles can lead to relationships that are richer and experiences that saturate our beings more deeply. Gratitude, too, isn't just a hashtag or a fancy diary; it's recognizing the mosaic of good pasted against the backdrop of existence, even amidst chaos.

Compiling narratives of our lives with a positive slant is like choosing the scenic route. Forget wrinkle creams and fountain-of-youth fantasies; owning and valuing our stories construct the scaffolding for a resilient, fulfilled self. Turns out, an autobiography penned with gusto is one that laughs in the face of time.

We mustn't forget the power of purpose. That fire-in-the-belly feeling that gets us out of bed in the morning is the ultimate elixir. It's fuel for living longer, not in the 'counting days' sense, but in terms of rich, vibrant, color-the-sky-with-your-dreams kind of days. Purpose propels us, and fulfillment sustains us; together, they weave the golden thread of a life well-lived.

Look, we all navigate the maze of life with different maps, but the 'X' marking the spot of longevity isn't just at the gym or the salad bar. It hovers in our mental atmospheres, in joy-spiked moments, and the quiet reflection of a sunset. In the end, it's the holistic blend of physical hustle and mindful harmony that spells out a life stretched to its fullest potential.

So let's bring it all home. When we lace up the sneakers of our psyche and hit the pavement of emotional fortitude, we're not just training for the marathon of a century. We're investing in quality miles, enriched by the thought that every moment is a treasure chest of vitality, a promise of tapping into the elusive, yet beckoning, infinity of life itself. The road to longevity is paved with the footprints of our mental and emotional journey as much as with sweat and leafy greens.

Building a support network for a longer, healthier life

So, let's chew on the often undervalued aspect of longevity: social networks. Not the digital kind that keeps your thumbs busy, but the real, flesh-and-blood connections that fuel your soul. Turns out, science has got your back on this and tells you, loud and clear, that your tribe, your people, your comrades-in-arms in the game of life play a monumental role in how long you'll stick around on this magnificent rock floating in space.

Imagine this – your support network, they're like your life's pit crew. They're there to get you back on track when you've blown a tire or to celebrate when you're leading the race. A heart-to-heart over coffee can do more than just perk up your day; these connections can literally add years to your life, strengthening your heart in the process. It's not some mystical, cosmic energy – although, let's face it, that concept has its charm. It's raw, biological truth – isolation isn't just uncomfortable, it's unhealthy.

We're social animals, and our brains light up like Vegas when we're surrounded by good company. It's not just about living longer; it's about living better. Those belly laughs, those shared tears – they're not just passing moments. They're life's elixir, a testament to our shared human experience that resonates deep within our cells, telling them, "Hey, life's pretty grand, let's keep this party going."

So how do you go about weaving this safety net that catches you when life hurdles lemons at lightning speeds? Start by being proactive. Reach out, connect, be genuinely interested in the souls that cross your path. It's not about the number of friends; it's the quality that counts. A handful of heartfelt relationships can be worth more than a thousand superficial acquaintances when it comes to your lifespan's scoreboard.

And hey, it's not just about the warm fuzzies. It's about the nitty-gritty benefits too. Your crew can sway you towards healthier habits, kind of like having a personal cheerleader for your daily salad instead of that double bacon cheeseburger. They're your accountability partners in the gym of life, coaxing you to lift a bit more weight, to push through that last rep of responsible choices, because man, it feels good to be strong, both inside and out.

Remember, this network isn't just about what you get; it's about what you give. It's a two-way street. Your zest for life can ignite a spark in others, and together, that blaze can light up the darkest of moments. It's about building a village where each person is a pillar, and collectively, you not only stand the test of time but you dance through it, with some killer moves to boot.

So, intersperse your quest for longevity with the pursuit of deep, meaningful relationships. Volunteer, join groups that align with your passions, strike up conversations without fear of awkward pauses. Learn to listen, really listen, and shine a spotlight on others, because in that glow, you'll both bask.

And for those moments when you're feeling like a solitary wolf, recall the howls of your kind in the distance. They're there, waiting, ready to remind you that you're part of a pack, a community, a network that's so intricately connected, they're the roots keeping your tree standing tall through the seasons of life.

One last thing. Let's not forget that heartache and struggle are part of the deal. They test the strength of your connections. You'll see who sticks around when the storms hit, who'll offer an umbrella, or who'll dance in the rain right beside you. These are the ties that bind tighter than most, weathered and worn, but undeniable in their durability.

In the grand kaleidoscope of life, extending our stay is not just a solo journey. It's a communal voyage, where each person you encounter adds a piece to your mosaic. So, invest in those pieces, cherish them, and watch how the picture they create helps you live not only a longer but an infinitely richer life. Let's not just aim for a lengthy existence, but a tapestry woven with threads of connection that turn surviving into thriving – together, we create the masterpiece of longevity.

Chapter 7: Beyond Mortality

If we let our imaginations leap beyond the constraints of our flesh and bones, we venture into a realm where 'forever' isn't just a fanciful notion—it's a legit endgame. What we're talking about isn't your garden-variety anti-aging cream or superfood elixir; we're tiptoeing into a world where humans tango with transhumanism, and the line between science fiction and reality gets blurrier than a vanishing horizon. Picture this: your consciousness, the whole chaotic, wonderful mess of thoughts and memories that make you, you—uploaded, downloaded, and outlasting the laptop you're reading this on. And a world without death? It's not merely about sidestepping the grave; it's reshaping the human experience with each pulse of a quantum computer. Inside every byte of data, there's a whisper of eternity, and we're here scratching our heads, pondering the implications, ethical mazes, and existential riddles of a universe that might just let us thumb our noses at the grim reaper.

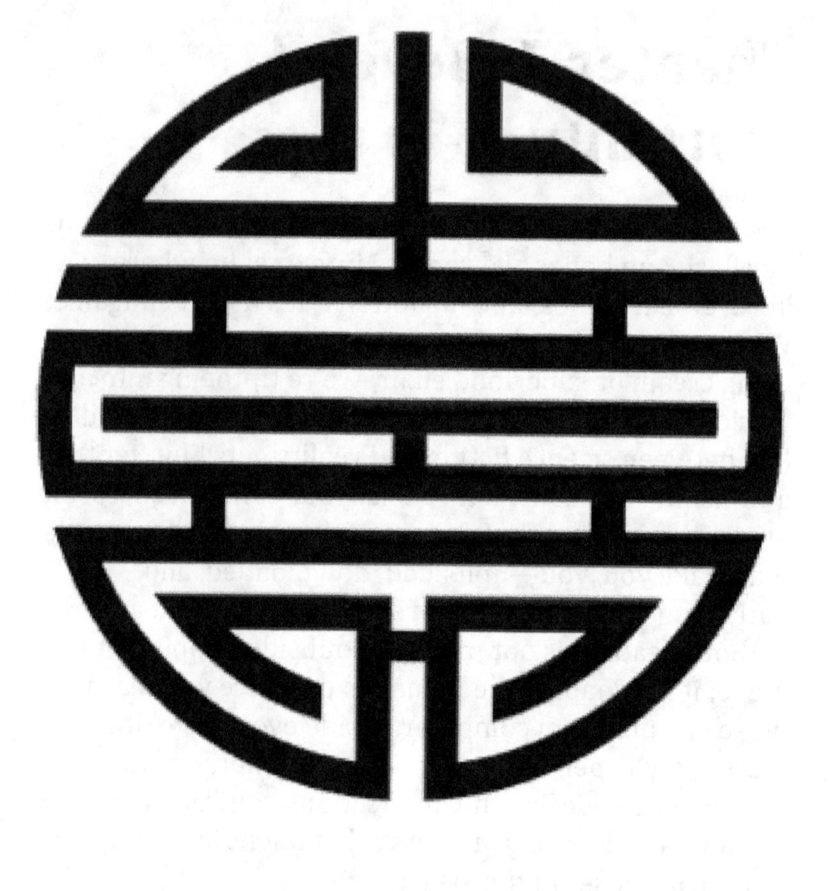

Exploring Concepts of Transhumanism and Post-Humanism

So we've journeyed through the biology of aging, optimizing mind and body, and looked at the ethical conundrums of chasing eternal life. Let's venture into some mind-bending ideas that really kick the door down on what it means to be human. Think transhumanism and post-humanism—an incredible, perhaps inevitable, and certainly controversial arc in our pursuit of dancing cheek-to-cheek with immortality.

Transhumanism is that next level where we're not just sprucing up the human condition—we're transcending it. Imagine enhancing your cognitive abilities so you're smart enough to make Einstein scratch his head. Or getting fitted with bionic limbs that would put Olympic athletes to shame. It's this belief that we can, and maybe should, augment our biological bodies to cope with challenges ahead and maybe to take our place among the stars.

But hit the pause button—how does becoming 'more than human' strike you? There's that cocktail of excitement and ethical vertigo. Because, let's be real, tweaking our genes and merging with machines straddle the line between sci-fi fantasy and a potential future that's tech-savvy utopia or dystopia in disguise.

Post-humanism takes a bit of a detour. It's less about upgrading the hardware and more about questioning the very concept of what humans are, and ultimately, what we could become. It's that theoretical playground where traditional notions of humanity get tossed in the blender with cultural, philosophical, and technological insights.

Are we defined by our limitations, or can we reframe the narrative of human destiny?

For instance, take the way technology is practically knitted into our daily lives. We've got the world's knowledge in the palm of our hand, and yet, we're just scratching the surface. Imagine if your memory, your experiences, and what makes you 'you' could be digitized. No, it's not the stuff of overnight ponderings—it's a serious conversation gaining traction as we speak.

The brain is complex, sure—the ultimate enigma wrapped in a riddle, smothered in mystery sauce. But what if we could untangle that complexity and understand it so well that we could recreate consciousness itself? That's the ticket to a different dimension of existence, where flesh and blood may be optional, and our digital selves could be shooting the breeze on some server for as long as we'd like them to.

Now, don't think this is all roses and sunshine. There's the gritty side where we need to ask tough questions. What does it mean to be human if you can live for centuries, with abilities that we today can only dream of? How will we grapple with consciousness that's not anchored to a beating heart or a breathy sigh?

Dive deeper, and we come across the idea of 'the singularity'—that moment when artificial intelligence surpasses human intelligence, potentially rendering us obsolete. Talk about an existential crisis on an epic scale. Do we then become the architects of a new species that'll look at Homo sapiens as a quaint, distant ancestor? The awesome potential and peril of these concepts need to stew in the collective consciousness; that's for sure.

In this grand pursuit of Beyond Mortality, aren't we really searching for meaning in life, even if it stretches indefinitely? Whether we choose to hack our biology, upgrade our bodies, or digitize our souls, beneath all that tech and possibility, there's the timeless quest to understand who we are and who we might become. These concepts are not just futurist dreams; they're intensively human narratives that continue to evolve, just like us.

Embrace these ideas, question them, wrestle with them—they're as important as they are astonishing. Transhumanism and post-humanism are not just topics for debate but manifestations of our unyielding desire to explore the potential of human creativity and resilience. As we stretch the boundaries, as long as we keep our ethical compass close, we're on a journey that's as audacious as it is profound.

The potential for uploading consciousness and digital immortality

Imagine for a moment a world where the essence of who you are—your memories, your thoughts, your personality—could be transferred onto a digital platform. This is the crux of the consciousness uploading debate, the digital equivalent of capturing your soul in a bottle. Some folks compare it to hitting the save button on a document that just happens to contain the entirety of your mental self. Now, there's something to chew on, isn't there?

As we dive headfirst into this watershed moment in human evolution, we're not just tickling the edges of science fiction anymore. This realm pulls together threads from neuroscience, computer science, philosophy, and maybe a hint of magic, for good measure. We're talking about a digital copy of the mind that could, theoretically, live on indefinitely. It's a form of digital immortality that has science junkies and philosophers alike scratching their heads in equal measures—and perhaps a little bit of exhilaration.

The idea hinges on the fact that every neuron, every electric zip and zap in your brain could be mapped and replicated in a computer system. It's a high-stakes game of connect-the-dots, where the prize is an eternal life of bytes and bits. But it's complex, right? Our current technology is like using a kiddie pool when we need an ocean. There's a daunting gap between what we want to achieve and the tools available.

Yet, the train of progress chugs along. We've seen astonishing breakthroughs in artificial intelligence that often make us pause and ponder the very nature of human intelligence. If we can create a machine that learns, adapts, and reasons, it's not such a giant leap to wonder about encoding the electric dance of our thoughts into a silicon brain.

But wait a second, let it simmer. The implications of this are staggering and not just on a personal level. What does this mean for our humanity, our society? Is it ethical to have a digital alter-ego eternally chattering away on a server farm somewhere?

If somehow we do manage to translate the neuro-symphony into code, we then face the mother of all philosophical conundrums. Would this digital you be 'you' in any real sense? Is the echo of a laugh or the shadow of a frown enough to preserve the essence of a lived life? This copy might have your wit, your knowledge, maybe even your penchant for late-night tacos, but can it capture your hopes, dreams, and fears? These are questions without easy answers, and they're very much still up for debate.

Even so, the potential perks are hard to dismiss. Consider the possibility of being free from the fragility of flesh and bone. This 'you' wouldn't age or fall ill. It could theoretically learn and grow without the limits of biology. After all, an algorithm doesn't need to sleep, eat, or take a vacation (though, what a digital entity would do on a vacation poses a rather amusing question).

On the flip side, the notion of digital immortality taps into deep-seated fears of obsolescence—a future where the organic human could become irrelevant. It's a theme you find plastered across dystopian fiction, but it's no longer a mere storytelling trope. Will the center hold, or are we spinning toward a reality where human consciousness becomes just another asset, potentially subject to hacking, manipulation, or endless replication?

The bridge to forever isn't built yet, but the blueprints are being sketched in boardrooms and laboratories right now. It's a dizzying landscape where myth and reality intermingle, and it's as fragile as it is fantastic. The potential is there, almost within our grasp, like a strange fruit hanging just above our heads. Will we jump to grab it? And if we do, can we handle the fall if the branch breaks?

While you chew on these thoughts, consider this: The quest beyond mortality, via the portal of digital consciousness, writes a new chapter in the age-old story of human ambition. It's a journey as perilous as it is wondrous, as daunting as it is inspiring, and ultimately, it will test the full measure of our intellect, our ethics, and our desire to endure.

Considering the implications of a world without death

Pause for a moment and consider a world that's transcended that final curtain call we know as death. What happens when 'The End' isn't so terminal after all? It's a head-spinner, isn't it? The ramifications of a deathless society ripple out in all directions, touching ethics, society, and the very earth we walk upon. So, let's pull on that thread and unravel some of these implications, from the microcosm of individual existence to the macrocosmic impact on our planet.

Imagine the personal journey. With no endpoint staring you down, what's your rush? Would you still feel that burn to achieve, to connect, to love with the same fervor? Perhaps the meaning of accomplishment and relationships would evolve, morphing into something less about scarcity of time and more about the richness of experience. We'd be in it for the long haul, and that could shift our values in ways we can't even fathom from our mortal perch.

But let's pivot and think about the population. It's already ballooning with the finite lives we lead. A world without death nudges us into territory that's hard to map. Our blue marble has its limits. Resources like space, food, and water are not a bottomless well. The balance between birth and death maintains some semblance of equilibrium. Disrupt that, and you've got to wonder, how do we manage the tension between sustaining life and sustaining a life worth living?

Let's not gloss over the societal shifts. I'm talking about the potential stagnation in cultural evolution. Traditionally, change is powered by the new perspectives each generation brings. If the old guard never passes, how does that dynamic change? Do we settle into an unyielding status quo or does innovation thrive, fueled by centuries of accumulated wisdom?

Also, chew on this: the nature of risk would transform. Would we play it safer, knowing we have all the time in the world to lose? Or does the thought of an endless existence embolden us to take leaps we'd never consider if life were fleeting? Each choice becomes part of an infinite web, rather than a finite path.

Then, there's the question of equity. Let's be real, the key to unlock death's door would likely be expensive, at least initially. Would immortality become the ultimate divider, a resource clung to by those with the means, while the rest watch their potential for eternity slip by? The societal divide could grow into a chasm with the haves holding the elixir of life and the have-nots relegated to the ephemerality of the past.

And speaking of the past, what about history? Without death, the significance of our narratives gets weird. When you can literally live through the consequences of actions taken centuries ago, does history become a never-ending story with evolving plots and subplots instead of clear lessons and conclusions?

But then think about love. Would eternal life cheapen it, or might it become the ultimate playground for the heart? Lifelong partnerships could span hundreds of years. Yet with an ever-expanding network of interactions over endless time, does love become an infinite variable, harder to pin down, yet richer in its complexity?

Moral and ethical implications abound as well. The sanctity of life becomes a whole new ballgame when life is unending. Our entire legal and moral framework, built around the bounds of a life that inevitably concludes, would need a serious overhaul. The existential questions of purpose and fulfillment would echo in a canyon of eternity, demanding answers we've never had to formulate before.

Finally, contemplate the impact on the human spirit. There's something to be said for the way the specter of death adds poignancy to life. Without that impetus, would the human experience become a plateau of contentment or a dull ache of monotony? The zest that comes from the fleeting nature of existence might be replaced with a yearning for the profound that only finitude provides.

As we orbit around these thoughts, remember that they're grounded in both imagination and inevitability. The course is uncharted, and the stakes are sky-high. This conversation isn't just cerebral—it's a peek into a possible future that challenges our perceptions and pokes at the very fabric of what it means to be alive in this universe. As we inch closer to the possibility of a deathless age, it's pivotal that we scrutinize the horizon with both caution and curiosity.

Chapter 8: Spiritual and Cultural Perspectives

Peering into the rich tapestry of spiritual beliefs and cultural narratives, we uncover a mosaic of insights about the eternal. It's almost like a dance, twirling through vibrant traditions where immortality isn't just a fleeting wish but a cornerstone—think river of life, reincarnation, nirvana. We're talking centuries, millennia even, of grappling with the meaning of existence, the finality of death, and the allure of what lies beyond. Every culture, every epoch adds a different hue to this portrayal of immortality, each with its unique signature etched in the collective consciousness. And here we are, painting our own strokes on this ever-evolving canvas, questioning how these age-old perspectives can mesh with our modern quest for longevity. Like a whispered legend passed down through generations, these spiritual and cultural lenses shape our understanding and inform the ways we seek to extend the bounds of life. Whether it's finding solace in the promise of an afterlife or charting a purpose-filled path in anticipation of an endless tomorrow, this chapter dives deep into the heart of what it means to search for this elusive, tantalizing forever.

Immortality in Religious and Spiritual Traditions

Let's face it, the human heart has always harbored a secret chambers for the eternal, a sort of inner sanctuary where the idea of living forever seems as natural as the cycle of day and night. And where does this yearning shine most brightly if not in the tapestry of religious and spiritual traditions woven through time? These concepts are as diverse as the believers who cherish them and often form the cornerstone of meaning and purpose in existence.

Dive into any major faith and you'll find immortality etched in its core. Take, for example, the ancient Egyptians with their Book of the Dead, a guidebook for the afterlife, making sure pharaohs and common folks alike could navigate the complexities of eternity. The Egyptians weren't playing around; they took their immortal afterlife seriously, with mummification as a physical testimony to their beliefs.

Swing over to Eastern philosophies and you're dealing with a whole different ballgame, where the goal isn't so much to live forever in the same form, but rather to escape the cycle of death and rebirth. In Hinduism and Buddhism, the soul isn't trying to become immortal; it's looking to reach a state beyond suffering, beyond the toil of mortality itself. The pursuit of Moksha or Nirvana is the ultimate spiritual touchdown, the dissolution of the self into the cosmic ocean where time and death are mere ripples on the surface.

Then there's Christianity, where immortality is pretty much the endgame of the faith. The promise of eternal life through belief in Jesus Christ is the central narrative running through the whole script and it's a potent concept that's shaped the Western world for millennia. To be saved is to be granted access to everlasting life, where death is but a doorway to a grander existence.

Islam also holds immortality at its heart but emphasizes the merits earned through a life lived in accordance with God's will. Paradise isn't a given; it's a well-deserved reward for the faithful, an eternal garden where the tribulations of life are replaced with peace and divine presence. And you better believe the stakes are high because the flip side, separation from God, carries its own kind of eternal weight.

Then there's the idea of reincarnation, which puts an interesting spin on the whole immortality gig. Instead of banking on a one-way ticket to an eternal realm, faiths like Sikhism, Jainism, and again, Hinduism and Buddhism, see the soul on a kind of cosmic do-over loop. The soul doesn't die; it simply sheds its earthly suit and slips into a new one, carrying the karmic baggage from life to life until it sorts itself out.

Even outside the formal realms of global religions, indigenous and tribal traditions harbor rich notions of immortality. Many Native American beliefs, for example, speak to the enduring interconnection between the living, their ancestors, and the natural world, a seamless web that death can't cut. An individual's spirit continues as a part of the whole, a comforting and grounding belief that ties one to the land and the lineage.

Of course, with all these varied perspectives on immortality, one has to get into the thick of it and ask, "What's the common thread?" It seems that, regardless of the flavor of faith, there's a consensus that what we see isn't all there is. There's more to the story than biology, more to the universe than physics and chemistry. It's as if all these traditions are tapping into a shared intuition about the human experience—a foundation of hope that there's something more beyond the final breath.

What's mind-boggling is the impact these immortal ideologies have had on civilizations. They influence law, culture, morality, and even drive scientific inquiry. Think about it; the desire to leap over the mortal coil is the jet fuel for so much of human endeavor, sparking explorations into medicine, space, and the human psyche.

Jumping into this conversation can get deep and sometimes a little controversial—there are skeptics who'd argue it's all wishful thinking, a human-made salve for the existential angst that comes with being aware of one's mortality. Yet, this doesn't diminish the fact that the concept of immortality is a powerful force in the human narrative, one that's driven us, comforted us, and challenged us in countless ways.

In essence, religious and spiritual traditions around the globe offer us a multicolored lens through which we can view our visceral longing for immortality. They're not just about what happens after we shuffle off this mortal coil; they're an invitation to reflect on the here and now, challenging us to live our lives in echo of the eternal. And one can't help but wonder, what does this enduring quest for life beyond death tell us about our potential, about our very nature as curious, soulful travelers on this shared journey of life?

Cultural attitudes towards life, death, and the afterlife

Roll around in this thought for a second: cultures all over the map have been toying with ideas about what it means to really live, die, and shuffle off this mortal coil since forever. When we pause and dig into these beliefs, it's like a kaleidoscope of perspectives shaping not only our values but our very pursuit of life extension.

Consider how in some corners of the world, life is seen as a brief spark – brilliant and intense but always at the mercy of the wind. In these cultures, death's not an end but a stepping stone, part of a journey where the soul takes center stage. The afterlife, then, isn't a gloomy, dreaded threshold but more like a reunion, a celebration, or even a cosmic do-over in places where reincarnation is the ticket.

Then there's the polar opposite vibe, where death is as final as the last page of a book, and that's okay. For folks with this outlook, it's all about jam-packing as much as they can into the now, giving the life they've got everything they've got. And their afterlife? If it's out there, it's not their focus; they're too busy sculpting their legacies in real-time.

Sashay through history and you'll see towering pyramids, elaborate burial tombs, and ancestor worship telling us that once upon a time (and still, in places), honoring the dead was as much about keeping them close as it was fearing what happens if you don't. But even then, these practices were all wrapped up in the hope of something beyond – another life, an immortal journey, or a spirit world where the party never stops.

Fast forward, and you've got the modern cocktail of skepticism, science, and spirituality making the convo about what's next all the more intoxicating. Are we matter temporarily conscious or eternal beings slumming it in the physical? Is there a scoreboard somewhere tallying our deeds, or is it more about the connections we make and the footprint we leave behind?

It's wild how much this stuff weaves into the morality of living forever, isn't it? I mean, if we start cracking the code on sticking around indefinitely, don't these beliefs become our compass for navigating those uncharted waters? Whether we're talking societal norms, personal ethics, or just the way we embrace our daily grind, it seems like our cultural lens on death and what follows is about to get a serious workout.

Think about it – an existence where funerals might become more like bon voyage parties because we might see the guest of honor again someday, digitally or in the flesh. And the afterlife, well, it could transform into an optional excursion, an add-on package for the life well survived. The way we mourn, remember, and move on is in for a revolution.

Just imagine for a sec how a change in the mortality game plan ripples through everything. If you're eyeing a forever-type scenario, does the bucket list just become the list? Do our life goals stretch out as long as those fabled Greek gods and their never-ending dramas? And heaven, hell, reincarnation, Nirvana – how do these concepts evolve as life extension shifts from sci-fi to just plain sci?

Okay, take a beat here. No matter where you stand – eyeing the afterlife with anticipation or shrugging it off as life's post-credits scene – there's no denying we're all part of a narrative that's bigger than any one of us. In this story, cultural attitudes about the big three – life, death, and whatever lies beyond – are more than traditions or philosophies; they're the raw materials for shaping our futures.

Sure, grappling with the idea of living on might shake the foundations of what's come before. But isn't that the point? As we skirt the edge of this new frontier, we can't help but bring along the ghosts of histories past, melting them down, forging new insights, and maybe, just maybe, learning how to live like we never have to say goodbye.

Finding meaning and purpose in the context of eternal life

When you stare down the possibility of an endless horizon of tomorrows, something curious happens. The questions of 'why' and 'what's the point' echo a little louder in the caverns of the soul. Because, here's the kicker - with the prospect of eternal life waving at us from the future like a distant relative, we're not just talking about adding a few more years. We're talking about rewriting the script on human purpose.

It's fascinating, isn't it? Throughout history, various cultural and spiritual systems have sketched life as a fleeting journey towards an end. A final destination, be it heaven, reincarnation, or some form of afterlife, gave life shape and meaning. But what if the endpoint keeps moving? What if it fades completely? We find ourselves back at the drawing board, redrafting the purpose of life if it's no longer to live well in preparation for death.

Consider the weight of legacy. Till now, leaving a mark for future generations was a drive for many. Build, create, influence, so your name stands the test of time. That's poetic, sure, but when time stretches indefinitely, does the concept of legacy lose its luster? What would a life inundated with perpetual tomorrows look like? Would you write a book, paint a portrait, sculpt a statue when you've got an eternity to tweak and perfect? Maybe it's the process, the act of creation that we'd have to find solace in, not the finished product.

And let's not forget the wild card in the pack - boredom. Imagine the challenge of staying hungry for new experiences when you have unlimited time on your hands. It's one thing to backpack across Europe with a sense of urgency, each day precious, each experience a pearl on the string of life. But with eternity, does the string just... keep going? No beginning, no end, just an endless loop of beads that might start to look and feel the same?

There's an underlying beat to this train of thought, a rhythm that dictates a search for purpose in self-growth and learning. If you're going to live forever, why not master every musical instrument? Learn every language, read every book, and understand every philosophy? The sheer magnitude of the potential for self-improvement boggles the mind. But, do centuries of self-improvement lead to enlightenment or just to a more sophisticated version of existential angst?

Then there's the concept of connection. The people around us, our relationships - they often act as compasses for our purpose. Eternity demands an expanded view of community and love. Maybe the soulmate concept gets challenged. Could you really have just one perfect match for eternity? Or perhaps commitments would become more about the journey shared, rather than the destination reached. Think about it. With limitless life spans, you could witness the evolution of societies, relationships, and love itself.

It all seems to circle back to now—the present. The beauty in fleeting moments that seems magnified by their impermanence may need to be rediscovered in a world where those moments never cease. It's hard to grasp, almost paradoxical, but maybe looking at eternity through the lens of spirituality suggests a call to live each moment as if it were both the first and the last.

So, within this eternal paradigm, meaning and purpose might evolve from being goalpost-oriented to being ever-present, dynamic conceptions. We would perhaps focus less on the 'what' and 'where' we're aiming for and more on the 'how' we're existing. Culturally, the collective narrative may shift from one of aspiration to be remembered, to one of living in a state of perpetual legacy - where every action is part of the ongoing story of humanity.

In a way, an eternal life strips us back to the bare roots of existence, to the questions that have teased philosophers for centuries. It asks us to consider, deeply and without the safety net of an end, what it means to be human. Perhaps, in this conversation between the past and the limitless future, we might just find the extraordinary – a tapestry of meaning woven from the threads of infinite tomorrows.

Eternal life stretches the canvas of existence further than we've ever had to contemplate. And, while it's mind-warping, it's not entirely out of reach. It's about anchoring into the depth of experience, finding purpose in perpetual growth, and redefining what it means to create and to connect. There's an art to finding meaning, and perhaps, it's an art we are just beginning to sketch in the context of an eternal life.

Chapter 9: Challenges and Risks

Diving headfirst into the taboo, this chapter isn't just about the sparkle and the allure of ticking clocks that refuse to wind down—it's about the gritty, sand-in-the-eyeballs truth of thumbing our noses at mortality. We're zooming in on the hurdles, the Kindly Ones snapping at the heels of those dizzy on ambrosia, the stuff that keeps you up at night—what about overpopulation, resource depletion, or the nightmarish scenarios where 'forever' isn't as shiny as it sounded in the brochure? Immortality is sexy until it's not, until you're stuck in a loop, or when societies fracture under the weight of generation upon generation vying for their piece of the pie. There's a balance to strike, between the siren call of endless tomorrows and the cold splash of reality, about managing not just personal eternity but a collective future that's brimming with more than just quantities of years, one that's sustainable, equitable, and frankly, worth sticking around for. That's what we gotta unpack, here amongst the celluloid dreams of digits that never stop counting and the cold hard dirt that says, 'Hey, remember me?'

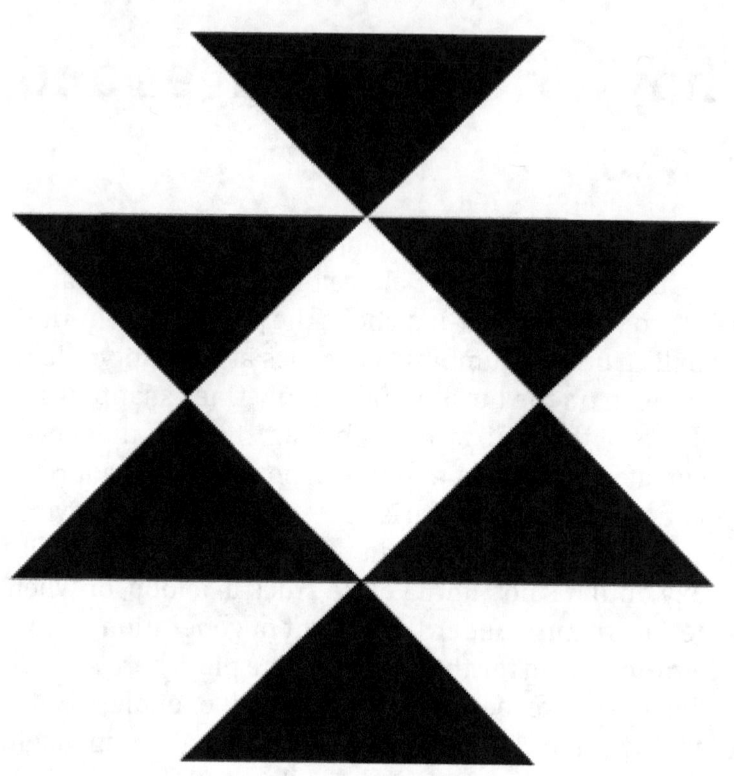

Potential drawbacks and challenges of living indefinitely

Tackling the beast of immortality is kind of like grabbing onto the tail of a dragon. It's thrilling, yeah, but what the heck do you do if you actually catch it? Imagine a life where age becomes just a number with an infinity symbol next to it. But living indefinitely? It's not all rainbows and butterflies. Let's dissect some of the heavier bricks in that load.

First off, think about the social fabric, a delicate piece of art really. We've spun this society with threads of beginnings, middles, and ends. But pull on the thread of eternity and everything could unravel. Families could stretch generations wide, and at some point, you'd have great-great-great-great (insert a hundred more 'greats') that you have to track at family reunions. Relationships could lose their urgency, their spice because "forever" suddenly really means forever. Think about it—would you rush to make amends or take that trip of a lifetime if you had all the time in the world? And let's not even start on pension plans; they'd be out the window along with the concept of retirement.

Then there's the almighty dollar—or yen or euro. The economy, bubbling and simmering with life cycles, could stall if everyone just keeps hanging around. Jobs could fill up, innovation might stutter because let's face it, a lot of great ideas come from fresh minds that haven't been jaded by, say, two centuries of "been there, done that." Plus, would you really be motivated to hustle if you knew you had an eternity to earn? The drive to achieve could sputter out without the time crunch.

On to resource management. We've only got one planet, and she's already sending us invoices for overuse. With an ever-lasting populace, we're looking at a full-blown sustainability crisis on steroids. We're talking food, water, energy, space—these are finite, even if we're not.

And let's talk personal growth. It's painful, messy, and beautiful. But it's fueled by that ticking clock, the knowledge that we're here for a good time, not a long time. When you're looking mortality in the eye, you're inspired to evolve, change, and reflect. Would we have the same drive to improve ourselves if we didn't have the pressure of a looming end? There's a chance that we might just get stuck in the perpetual loop of okayness.

That brings us to the psychological whirlpool. The human mind is an intricate mechanism that runs on balance—a cocktail of chemicals and experiences. It's tuned to handle the human lifespan as we know it. How would your brain—and mine—handle centuries? Just think about the backlog of memories, the potential for eternal grief as you outlive loved ones who choose the natural path or lost to accidents, or the Groundhog Day effect of an endless life. We might just end up with a societal case of existential ennui.

Now, idle hands and all that jazz—if we're not aging, what's to keep us from falling into a pit of boredom? Humans thrive on challenges, obstacles, and goals. Longevity could strip away the race against time that fuels innovation and personal achievements. What happens to progress when the whole concept of a "lifetime" is thrown out the window?

Speaking of windows, variety is the one that lets the light in. Diversity in experiences, perspective, and thoughts is what keeps life interesting. But if we're living indefinitely, do we eventually become homogenized clumps drifting through the epochs? Variety might not just be the spice of life; it might be the very essence of it.

Mortality has this way of making us peer into the abyss and ponder the big questions. It's a profound force that shapes philosophy, art, literature, and basically all the soul-stuff that makes life feel meaningful. So, if we take death out of the equation, what happens to our drive to understand the universe, ourselves, and our place in the grand scheme of things? Our art, our music, our stories—are they as deep and vibrant without the shadow of the end coloring them?

Finally, we circle back to the planet—our shared cradle and grave. An immortal population would place unprecedented strains on Earth. We're already scrambling to figure out how to deal with climate change, habitat loss, and more with the population we've got. What happens when no one exits stage left? There's also the basic biology of evolution, which relies on birth, mutation, and yes, death, to keep the train chugging. When we hit the brakes on that, how do we avoid stalling out as a species?

Let's face it: we've got a full plate chewing on mortality, so tacking on eternity is kind of like grabbing another plate when we haven't finished the first. It's enticing, no doubt, but with all these caveats, we've got to ask ourselves if we're really up for it. Sure, peering into the abyss is frightening, but it's also where we find the grit, the joy, and the sheer thrill of being alive. Living indefinitely? It might just be that the beauty of this world is that nothing lasts forever—not even life.

Addressing Societal and Environmental Impacts of Extended Lifespans

Imagine living in a world where the fountain of youth isn't just a mythical tale but a palpable reality. As we push the boundaries of science and uncover new ways to add more candles to the birthday cake, we can't help but wonder what ripples these extended lifespans will create in the pond of our society and environment. Let's wade into these waters slowly, shall we?

With people sticking around for what might seem like an extra act in life's play, the stage is set for overcrowding and generational pileup. You've probably already felt that sense of encroaching space at a family reunion or in a bustling city street. Now, crank that up a notch. More people can mean heavier strains on social systems designed for shorter life arcs – healthcare, pensions, social security. What happens when retirement isn't just a few decades, but a few generations?

And let's not even get started on the job market. Who's going to step aside for the sprightly new grads when everyone's holding onto their desk chairs for dear life? We'd need a new harmony, a symphony of age and youth blending in the workforce. Without it, we're just setting up for a generational showdown at the job fair.

But it's not just a game of musical chairs in office cubicles. There's a bigger picture we can't ignore. Our blue marble, Earth, she's carrying the weight of our ambitions and our growing numbers. Each person is a consumer, an eater, and, let's face it, a polluter. More mouths to feed means more farmland, more forests turning into strip malls. The environmental balance could go haywire unless we find a more sustainable way to dance this dance of longevity.

Now, think about inequality for a second. It's like we're at a buffet where some folks are filling their plates to the brim while others are getting crumbs. Extended lifespans might exaggerate this, creating a world where the rich get to enjoy endless summers while the less fortunate can barely make it through the winter of their years. How's that for a divided society?

But let's not just doom-scroll through the what-ifs. People are resourceful; they innovate, create, find loopholes in problems as stubborn as a jar lid that won't budge. So maybe we could create cities that rise to the sky or burrow into the earth, find alternate food sources that leave a softer footprint, or even colonize the stars. Humanity's ability to adapt is admittedly pretty impressive.

Discussions around 'fairness' come to the fore, too. Who gets to sip from this elixir of life extension? Can we really stomach a world where immortality becomes the ultimate luxury item? And let's not gloss over our own psychological ballet—how do we deal with the persistence of memory, love, loss, and the evolving self, if the self just keeps on going and going?

Here's a nugget to chew on—extended lifespans could actually prod us into becoming better stewards of our planet. Think about it. If you know you're going to be around for the sequels to your favorite movie saga that's expected to roll out over the next century, you might be more invested in keeping the theater clean, right? A longer life could mean more people taking a long-term interest in sustainability and conservation. We could witness a shift in mindset from 'not in my backyard' to 'not in my many, many years.'

It's a tangled web, no doubt. But remember, building this prolonged future is not just about adding years to life, but life to those years. It's not about outsmarting time; it's about enhancing the quality of existence in every tick and tock. We've got our work cut out for us to make sure society and environment don't fall to the sidelines in this march towards longevity.

So while the tapestry of eternal life is weaved with threads of innovation and hopes of an ageless tomorrow, let's keep our eyes peeled for those frays—those inklings of societal and environmental impacts. And hey, let's work on threading the needle with solutions that strengthen, rather than unravel, the beautiful, complex fabric we all share.

Balancing the Desire for Immortality with the Realities of Existence

Here we are, then, riding the crest of the wave that's been building since humans could first ponder their own existence — the wave of the dream of immortality. But let's not get carried away on that wave just yet. Balance, you see, is the name of the game when we're talking about the concept of living indefinitely. It's a tightrope walk above the stark realities of our mortal lives. Have you ever thought about what it really means to step out of the shadows of our own finitude?

Immortality stirs within us a flurry of emotions, doesn't it? There's the exhilaration of eternal youth, the hope of experiencing the future's wonders, and the desire to unravel every mystery of the universe. That's one rocking party that nobody wants to leave early. But at what point does the never-ending bash clash with the gentle rhythm of our earthly score?

Consider the environment: our beautiful sphere, resilient yet so fragile. We're already pushing her limits with our current lifespans. Imagine that but stretched out over centuries. There's a dilemma for you — the pursuit of everlasting life could mean outliving the planet that sustains us. It's like trying to have your cake and eat it too on a ship that's running out of supplies — it just can't sail on forever.

Then there's the social fabric that knits together our sense of humanity. Society as we know it is a dance of generations, each one stepping in and out to the tune of time. If nobody ever leaves the dance floor, how will the dance evolve? For the world to strive, we've got to keep it fresh with new thoughts, new dreams. Staying forever young in body is one thing, but staying forever adaptable in spirit, that's the real challenge.

Transitioning onto personal terrain, the landscape gets even trickier. Relationships, passions, goals — they all have their seasons, don't they? If you're sticking around indefinitely, how do you keep the fire burning in the hearth of your life? It's a heck of a thing to contemplate, enough to make you wonder if immortality might be the ultimate test of love, interest, and ambition.

Let's dive even deeper now. The essence of living — isn't it about growth, change, and ultimately, transformation? There's an argument that without an end, we might just lose our drive to make every moment count. It's the deadline, after all, that lights a fire under us, gets us moving, pushes us to make a difference. Could the secret sauce of life be its very impermanence?

Grapple with the ethics for a moment. The chance for extended life won't likely land on every doorstep at the same time. Who gets to sip from the fountain first? It's a moral minefield. Equality and immortality might just find themselves on opposite sides of the battlefield. It's crucial that we ensure that the moral compass guiding the ship stays true, encompassing all of humanity and not just a privileged few.

So, you see, the yearning for endless days comes wrapped in complex packages, handed from the realms of science, philosophy, and spirit. In our quest, we have to ask the tough questions. Are we seeking mere survival, or are we on a quest for a life brimming with meaning and purpose? The balance lies perhaps not in outrunning time, but in running with it, side by side, savoring each stride.

Picture it: a world straddling the line between mortality and a never-ending horizon. Would you, if given the chance, step across that line or would the very earth beneath your feet seem to shift, the sky above seem less infinite, the moments less sweet? Perhaps it is the looming whisper of an end that instills value in our times and tales.

We're pioneers on the frontiers of the possible and the imagined. But let's not forget to tread with care, considering the mosaic of implications each step brings forth. Living indefinitely isn't just a personal journey; it's a collective expedition filled with responsibility, wisdom, and above all, respect for the delicate dance of existence.

Chapter 10: The Future of Immortality

Time is a funny thing; we chase it, try to hold onto it, but it's always slipping through our fingers. Yet, here we are, on the cusp of turning the tables—imagine a world where the aged clock doesn't just slow, but halts, where the very essence of time becomes a companion rather than a thief. As our journey through the landscapes of timelessness inches toward the horizon, we're beckoned by the whispers of immortality that mingle with the steadfast march of progress. We've traversed the realms of nutrition, dissected the enigmas of the mind, and danced with the technologies that could one day stitch eternity into the human fabric.

And now, we find ourselves peering into the realms of possibility, where the fusion of ambition and innovation brews a potent elixir of everlasting life. The question isn't just 'can we?' but 'how will we?' navigate the brave new world where silver locks are but a choice. The unwritten chapter lies before us, threaded with the thrilling pulse of regenerative medicine, nanotechnology that whispers healing secrets to our cells, and the digital realms poised to cradle our consciousness. We stand at the crossroads, contemplating how the symphony of science will harmonize with the intrinsic yearning for infinity—an inquiry both exhilarating and humbling under the shadow of stars that have watched life's drama unfold across eons. What awaits is not just a new chapter in human history but a new epoch in the chronicle of existence itself.

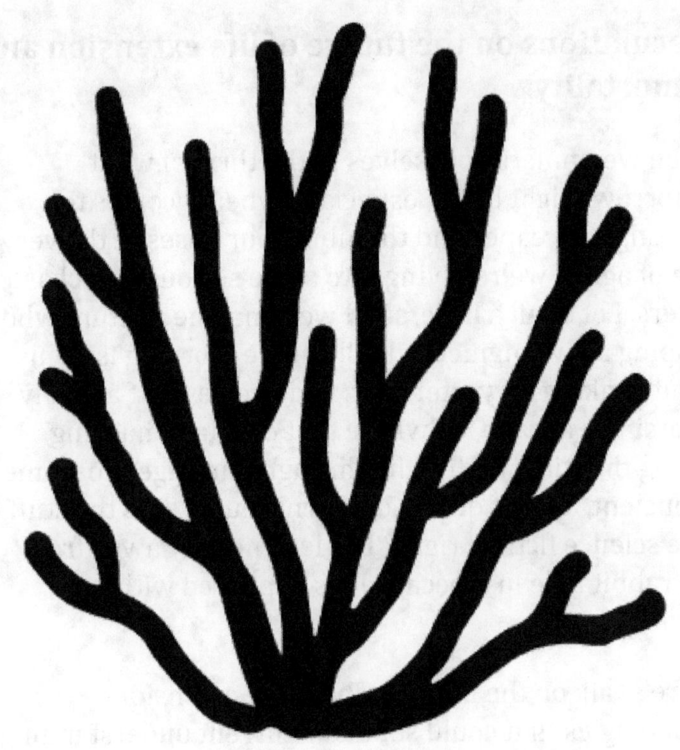

Speculations on the future of life extension and immortality

When we immerse ourselves in the thrill of what tomorrow might bring, especially when it comes to cheating the reaper and thumbing our noses at the very idea of aging, we're diving into some seriously uncharted waters. Let's sail a little, shall we? Imagine a future where popping a few engineered pills in the morning isn't just about shaking off yesterday's bad choices, but actually reversing a decade. Or where that constant, nagging feeling that time is slipping through our fingers becomes an ancient, almost quaint concern. Sounds like the stuff of pure science fiction, right? But let's not shy away from this rabbit hole just because it's peppered with unknowns.

There's talk on the horizon about life extension technologies that could send our current understanding of biology and longevity into a tailspin. We're not just tinkering at the edges of our lifespans; we're storming the fortress of mortality, armed with CRISPR gene editing and breakthroughs in nanotechnology that might one day repair our cells like tiny engineers. One day you might wake up, look in the mirror and see a version of yourself that's not only healthier but decades younger. Now, if that's not a wild wake-up call, I don't know what is.

And let's not forget about the mystical marriage of man and machine, the bionic convergence where our biology mates with artificial intelligence. Got a failing organ? Here's a synthetic replacement that's better than the original. Losing memories? Perhaps there will be an implant for that. It's like we could be walking into a real-life 'upgrade' station.

But this is where things get twisty. With immortality possibly dangling within our grasp, what does it even mean to live a good life? If you thought navigating your twenties was complex, imagine doing it for an eternity. The philosophical implications are staggering. Would we still cherish sunsets or the laughter of children if we knew they were experiences that could be had ad infinitum? As much as eternal life teases us with endless possibilities, it also throws us into a sea of existential questions without a lifeboat.

Let's take a breather and wheel back to the science for a sec. Some fiercely intelligent minds are now speculating that every part of our bodies could be regenerated, rejuvenated, or replaced. They're not crazy; they're just ahead of the curve. We may just be a few groundbreaking studies away from turning sci-fi dreams into concrete, injectable, wearable, livable realities. Heart giving out on you? Let's grow you a new one. Brain getting foggy? Tune it up with a neurostimulation device.

This brave, new world, however, doesn't come without its own bag of snakes. Extending life is one thing, but ensuring quality of life is another beast altogether. We'll need to balance our youthful vigor with a wisdom that doesn't come in pill form. Longevity begs for a life well-lived, not just a long one. And it's crucial that we don't forget the soulful side of existence, which makes life sparkle, even if we can technically live forever.

Let's also ponder the ripple effect. Imagine the shifts in global demographics, economies in turmoil as retirement ages become obsolete, resources stretching thin because, well, no one is bowing out. Say hello to new societal puzzles that we'll need to piece together, redefining family structures, careers, and maybe even love itself. If love is eternal, so could be our relationships—'til death do us part' could take on a whole new meaning, or no meaning at all.

When all is said and done, though, this relentless pursuit is about more than just staying alive. It's about what we do with that life. The search for immortality, in many ways, is the ultimate reflection of our human ambition, our tenacity, our refusal to accept the status quo. It's about aspiring to a future where our fates aren't written by the hands of time but authored by our own passion and ingenuity.

However outlandish it may seem, the future of life extension and immortality is creeping closer to today's science than yesterday's mythology. We'll keep pushing the boundaries, redefining what's possible, and, in the process, redefining humanity itself. So as we gear up for the thrilling, wild ride into this great unknown, let's keep our heads on straight, our hearts open, and our eyes peeled for the sunrise of a world where 'forever' might just be the new normal.

In the last dance of this section, let's not discard the thought of a world brimming with centenarians who look and feel like they're in their prime. It's a place where terms like 'aging gracefully' become archaic, where the phrase 'against the sands of time' is nothing but a reference to a fight we once believed was unwinnable. Yes, speculation indeed, but one that sows the seeds for a garden of immortality that we may one day walk through, wondering how we ever lived any other way.

The intersection of technology, science, and human ambition

Peering into the churning crucible where technology, science, and undying human ambition meld together, we're staring down the barrel of a concept so enthralling, it might as well be magic. But let's not kid ourselves, this isn't a tale of wands and wizards—this is real life, where every breakthrough feels like one step closer to unraveling the ancient riddle of immortality. So, what's at this fascinating crossroads?

Imagine a world where nanobots rove through your veins, repairing cells almost the moment they show signs of aging. Picture a future where our very genetic blueprint is tinkered with, not in the dark recesses of some sci-fi nightmare, but in the bright, promising labs of today, reshaping our destiny. We're on the cusp of fusing our biological beings with an arsenal of tech that could blast the concept of aging into oblivion. It's not just about living longer; it's about living better, richer, and with more gusto than we've ever dared to dream.

At this juncture, technology and science aren't just buddies; they're intertwined partners in a dance of progress. Genetic engineering? Check. Augmented reality for cognitive training? Check. AI that can predict your health trajectory and tweak it for the better? Double-check. It's a symphony where each note is a discovery or invention, and guess what—the maestro is human ambition. Always pushing, always striving, and let's face it, always a bit greedy for more days under the sun.

But pause for a sec and chew on this—beating aging is also about the sheer willpower to reach for what once seemed unattainable. It's like climbing a mountain, not because it's there, but because on the other side might just be the fountain of youth that's captivated our fantasies since the dawn of time. Each step up is another breakthrough, another possibility—maybe it's a pill, a gene therapy, or a consciousness upload into the cloud; the how isn't as important as the burning why.

Speaking of mountain climbing, let's not overlook our own wiring. We're basically hardwired for survival. Every cell in our body screams it, every beat of our heart confirms it. And now, we're taking that primal instinct and channeling it into a storm of innovation that might just redefine the human experience.

Maybe you're thinking, "Calm down, it's not all sunshine and roses." And you'd be right. This crossroads is also a cliff's edge, teetering over questions of morality, ethics, and the very fabric of society. But can't you just sense it? The vigor that comes with even the slimmest chance that we might break our biological bonds and step into the realm of the gods? It's intoxicating, and it's what keeps humanity clawing upwards, searching for the elusive key to an endless tomorrow.

The methods and machines we're devising aren't just cold steel and emotionless circuits—they're the offspring of curiosity and boldness. They're nurtured by the stories of Ponce de Leon, the myths of alchemy, and every person who ever wished upon a star for just one more day with a loved one.

At this intersection, we're not just scientists or tech wizards—we're poets and prophets, dreamers and doers. We're the kids who never stopped asking "what if" and "why not." So, as we stand at this electrifying confluence, with the power to potentially unlock eternity itself, it's not just the gears and gadgets that will lead the way. It's our defining human spark, that tempest of desire and drive that's blazed a trail through history and, if we play our cards right, might just light up the path to forever.

Now, let me level with you, diving into the future headfirst won't be without its belly flops. But since when has that stopped us? With every fiber of our being, we seek to transcend limits, to reach for the stars, literally and metaphorically. It's our next Everest, our moon landing, our crossing of the Rubicon—and in this quest for immortality, the very same attributes that make us undeniably human could be the launchpad to our greatest escapade yet.

The future of immortality isn't a certainty—it's a question mark, a painting unfinished, a story mid-sentence. But if one thing's for sure, this crossroads, this exhilarating nexus of technology, science, and raw, unfiltered ambition, isn't just a chance at more time. It's a challenge, a promise, and a journey we're wired to embark on. And what a ride it promises to be.

Envisioning a world where immortality is within reach

Imagine, if you will, a place where the ticking of the biological clock doesn't spell out an end but merely serves as a background rhythm to the symphony of life — enduring, perpetual. This isn't just some flight of fancy but a logical terminus we're careening toward, where mortality becomes optional, age just a number, life an infinite corridor of possibilities. Take a minute, dig into that — the notion of eons stretched out before you, not with the weariness of time but with the boundless vigor of youth.

What would you do with all that time? Would you finally pen the next great American novel, decode the mysteries of the universe, or simply bask in endless summers, every relationship unbounded by the tyranny of time? Picture the leaps in technology that make such questions more than a mental exercise. Biotechnology's no longer just a chapter in a science book; it's the architect sketching the blueprints of tomorrow.

Peering through the lens of possibility, genetic wonders brew in labs across the globe. Scientists splice and dice at the very twine of life, tweaking longevity genes as though they were strands of code in an open-source program. Meld this with the relentless progress in regenerative medicine, where one's own cells work as dutiful artisans, sculpting our organs anew, repairing the wear and tear that years have wrought.

Now don't get it twisted — immortality's not just about having an endless timeline. It's about quality, not just quantity. Think enhanced bodies, minds as sharp as knives forever, art and philosophy flourishing like never before, because let's face it, the brightest flames could burn so much longer, illuminating the path to an ever-expanding horizon of human achievement.

Consider the impact on wisdom, empathy, the maturation of societies that are no longer racing against a clock but rather strolling through eons, soaking in the experience. Wars and conflicts might become relics of an age when humans lived in the fast lane, life cheap because it was, in essence, short. In a long-life society, we might see an explosion of stability and foresight.

In truth, it's not just a matter of staying alive but staying alive well — keeping body and soul tethered in harmony. The canvas of life blooms with artistry when the fear of the final curtain call is erased. Remember, it's one thing to give someone a million years, it's another to fill those years with meaning that enriches not just the individual, but humanity as a whole.

Admittedly, the myriad streams of ethical and philosophical debates converge here: the allocation of endless time, the stratification of society, the very ecosystem we inhabit — will it shoulder the load? How do we mold a world where the old don't outstay the new but rather coexist, where wisdom threads through generations like a golden tapestry unmarred by the attrition of time?

Finding the path to immortality isn't just about breaking biological barriers. It's about spiraling upwards, transcending the known limits of human potential. It's about envisaging radically transformed cultural landscapes, where death and taxes are no longer the only certainties. It's about grappling with the idea that our saga may not have a final chapter, that the story keeps unravelling into uncharted territories of self and substance.

Peek into this envisaged future, the aroma of eternity in the air, the pursuit of passions and knowledge untethered. You might learn every language, help construct the spaceship meant to visit distant stars, participate in constructing a utopia — not once wondering if the hourglass is running low.

As we stand at the brink of this revolutionary epoch, let's hold onto our hats, not out of fear, but in homage to the winds of change, to a future where the twilight years need not dim, but rather herald in long, golden hours of potential fulfilled, humanity reborn in the glow of immortality's dawn.

Chapter 11: Epilogue: Embracing the Journey

As we close the cover on this exploration of time's tightrope, it dawns on us that the race towards immortality is more than a checklist of scientific breakthroughs, doses of wisdom, or extreme feats—it's an intricate dance of being and becoming. Life's cadence may push us towards the next big thing in longevity, but let's also soak in the here and now, shall we? It's about squaring off with our mortality, appreciating the grit and grace of the human experience, and finding an indomitable spirit that outlives the ticking clock. Accepting the undulating paths of our journey liberates us; it's the pulse in our veins, the thoughts coursing through our minds—this interwoven fabric of immediacy and infinity that makes us feel alive. And so, we stand on the precipice of the unknown, peering into the horizon with hearts swelling with the joy of possibility, acknowledging a future replete with promise yet honoring the profound simplicity of a single, well-lived moment.

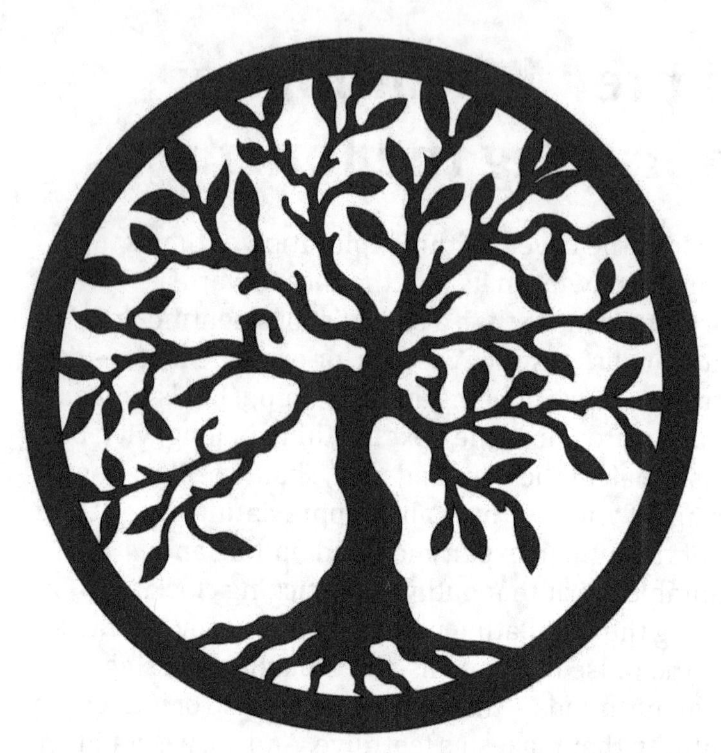

Reflecting on the quest for immortality and the meaning of life

As we journey through the winding path of existential thought and scientific discovery, it's essential to pause and ponder on the very nature of our pursuit of immortality. What drives this insatiable thirst for eternal life? It seems woven into our DNA, this relentless push against the natural order, this refusal to accept the boundary between existence and oblivion. We're wired to survive, sure, but why the leap towards forever? Maybe it's a fear of the unknown, of the great void that death implies, or perhaps, it's the love for life that fuels our desire to hold on ad infinitum.

The thought is perplexing, isn't it? Immortality, as a concept, stretches beyond the grasp of our mortal hands, and yet, we reach for it with everything we've got. Scientific advancements propel us forward, inching closer to what once was the domain of gods and myths. But let's be real—extending life indefinitely comes with a suitcase full of ethical, social, and philosophical dilemmas. Will we even recognize ourselves in this new age of humanity? It's like staring into the abyss and seeing the abyss stare back—exciting and unnerving all at once.

The endless search for the fountain of youth isn't just about dodging death. It's also about redefining what it means to live. Life's brevity gives it zest—the vibrant colors of sunrise, the depth of love's first kiss, the piercing pain of loss. They're all punctuated by the ticking clock. Yet, if that clock were to stop... would these experiences hold the same weight? Or would they blend into an eternal, indistinct horizon?

We ought to consider that perhaps, chasing after immortality is like chasing after the horizon. No matter how much we run, how much we optimize our bodies and minds, crunch our nutrition, and hack our biology, that line where the earth meets the sky remains out of reach. Could it be that the richness of life lies not in its length but in its content? The flavors we savor, the bonds we forge, the legacies we leave—a finite timeline might just be the canvas on which these elements can truly stand out.

It's funny, in a way. Here we are, taking on mortality like it's a challenge to conquer, a peak to summit. But with each step up the mountain, the air gets thinner, and we're reminded of our intrinsic human limits. Isn't it the climb itself that fills our lungs with fresh air, our hearts with fire? It's not about planting our flag on some eternal plateau; it's about the ascent—the people we meet, the knowledge we gain, the love we share.

Let's face it, immortality might turn out to be less about evading death and more about embracing life. Maybe it's this moment, right here, right now, that holds the ultimate value. It's bittersweet, to think we're here for just a blink in the universe's grand timeline. Yet, it's profoundly beautiful too. Within our ephemeral existence, we find the urgency to create, to explore, to love, and to learn.

Imagine, just for a moment, a world where death is not a certainty but a choice. How would that shift our view on what it means to be alive? It's like holding a book with infinite pages—you'd never feel the rush to turn the next page for fear of reaching the end. But isn't there a reason why stories have a final chapter, why songs have a closing note? There's a rhythm to life, a natural ebb and flow that shapes our collective and individual narratives. We may well extend the final note, but we can't forget the music that plays in between.

As we stand on the precipice of potential immortality, let's not lose sight of the very essence that makes life precious. Our quest for more time—whether obtained through technology, spirituality, or sheer human will—should not overshadow what we do with that time. The question isn't just "Can we live forever?" but "What kind of life do we want to lead?" Because, in the end, the value of our days isn't measured in the number of sunsets we've seen, but in the depth of experiences that each sunset represents.

In the dance with our destiny, we may find that the beauty of life is not in its potential for permanence, but in its profound temporality. Our impermanence gives us the context to strive, to cherish, and to change. So let's not just strive for a heartbeat that never stops; let's aim for a life that truly resonates with every beat. If immortality is on the horizon, let us approach it not as a runaway from death but as adventurers seeking to live each day with passion and purpose.

And so, as we close this chapter—whether it leads to another or it's the final word on our journey—let's live. Not for the sake of tallying years but for filling those years with laughter, tears, triumphs, and the vast spectrum of human experience. Immortality? Maybe it's not about conquering time but about making every moment count. After all, isn't a life well-lived the most timeless legacy of all?

Embracing the present moment while striving for a longer future

So here we stand at the precipice, gazing into the vast expanse of what may be an endless horizon. The journey has been extraordinary, hasn't it? Each step has unearthed a puzzle piece to the grand tapestry of extended life and maybe even immortality. Yet within this tapestry lies a vital thread, one that binds us to the here and now: the precious, irreplaceable present moment.

It's easy, amidst the excitement of scientific breakthroughs and the allure of age-defying marvels, to let the current slip like sand through tightly clenched fingers. But hold on a second—what are we racing towards if every heartbeat of today feels like a step out of sync? It's crucial, imperative even, to cherish this very instant, this breath, this heartbeat.

Capturing the essence of the present isn't about halting our stride towards a brighter tomorrow. No, it's quite the opposite. It's about infusing every step with intention, with passion, with the fullness of life that we're trying to extend. Every shared laugh, every sunset, every hug from a loved one—it's these moments that inject color into the otherwise monochromatic pursuit of longevity.

Pause for a moment. There's power in that—power in relishing the taste of your morning coffee, in feeling the warmth of the sun on your skin, in listening to the symphony of life that buzzes all around. Our journey towards greater sunsets, lengthier life spans, and eons of exploration must be rooted in the fertile soil of the now.

Sure, we're wired to seek tomorrow, to quest for a promised land of perpetual tomorrows. Yet, in chasing this dream, let's not forget that life—real, visceral living—happens today. Even as we ponder the potential to transcend our biological clocks, maintain a presence of mind that celebrates this minute, this second, with the same vigor we reserve for the next breakthrough on the horizon.

It's not about eschewing foresight or abandoning our ambition for a longer future. It's about marrying the pursuit with a mindfulness that amplifies our experience. Each breath is a gift, delivering the oxygen we're so hell-bent on savoring for eons. Isn't it ironic? In the end, it's the simplest things that we crave more of—more connections, more laughs, more love.

Embrace a dual mindset. One that is steadfast in its commitment to a future where age is but a concept, while simultaneously cultivating a profound appreciation for the transient tapestry that is the human experience. This duality is the fulcrum upon which a fulfilling life tilts—always stretching forward but firmly rooted in the effervescent and ephemeral 'now'.

As we widen our grasp to include the potentialities of an infinite existence, let's tighten our embrace around the day-to-day joys. The thing is, we're not simply after more time—we're after more life within that time. A paradox, perhaps, of wanting to live forever yet realizing the only forever we truly have unfolds in consecutive strings of now.

Strive, then. Strive for longevity, strive for vitality, strive for a future beaming with unexplored life. But let that striving be laced with a profound attachment to what surrounds us this very moment. For in this balance, we find the grace of a life well-lived—long or short, simple or awash with complexity. It's in the art of embracing the journey, step by step, breath by breath, that we truly understand the essence of immortality.

And when the sun sets on this chapter, on this exploration of what it means to defy time, may we each hold a heart full of present joys—memories that, irrespective of whether tomorrow comes, pronounce us infinite in the moments we've fully, wholly lived. This, perhaps, is the simplest yet most profound secret to a longer future. It's not just about quantity of years; it's about quality of moments, fiercely, tenderly alive.

Concluding thoughts on living a fulfilling and purposeful life, whether immortal or not

So, we've trekked through the vast and complex landscape of immortality—from the biology of aging to the edge of transhumanism. Yet, in the end, isn't it about the pursuit of living a life so rich and deep that whether we cease to exist tomorrow or a millennium from now becomes a secondary concern? It's the essence of being truly alive that captivates us, terrifies us, and ultimately defines us.

Living a purposeful life is like composing a symphony, where each day is a new note that contributes to the harmony. If we're just chasing the horizons of our lifespan without savoring the melodies of daily experiences, are we not just living on repeat, waiting for something to happen? It's not just about tacking on years; it's about infusing those years with quality, purpose, and connection.

If we're going to potentially live forever, then let's talk about what makes life fulfilling. It's those moments when you feel connected to something greater, when you're so absorbed in an activity that time falls away. It's the relationship that challenges and grows you, the project that ignites your passion, and the generosity that expands your heart. This is true richness, with or without immortality.

Nurturing the body is undeniably important. Our vessels carry us through this beautiful world, and treating them with respect through nutrition, exercise, and rest is a no-brainer. But we often forget that the non-tangible aspects of our lives—the laughter, the love, the leaps of faith—are just as vital for longevity. A balanced mind exudes a radiance that exercise alone can't sculpt into our spirits.

Let's also take a step back and ponder the ethical and philosophical conundrums we tackled in earlier chapters. What good is living forever if society crumbles under the weight of our collective existence? It's a balancing act between selfish and selfless—exploring the bounds of life extension while considering the ecological and social ramifications. A truly purposeful life is cognizant not just of personal desires, but also of the well-being of others and our planet.

Then there's the cultural and spiritual dimension—how our understanding of immortality shapes our worldviews. Wrapped in the spiritual tapestry of our lives are the threads of eternal existence, rebirth, and transcendence. These are not ideas to be shelved until our twilight years; they are concepts to be woven into the everyday fabric of our lives, guiding our actions and framing our intentions.

Are we really prepared for the challenges and risks of living indefinitely? Or, paradoxically, do these uncertainties motivate us to dive headfirst into the now—to embrace every morning's sunrise, every shared secret, and every dream pursued with audacity? Maybe it's the very presence of an ending that intensifies our commitment to living fully.

The future, as always, is a fog we peer into with a mixture of hope and anxiety. The seamless blend of technology and biology beckons a horizon filled with potential, but uncertainty is the shadow that trails every leap of progress. Amidst such speculations, the only truth we have is the present moment, the realness of now, and the choices we make in pursuit of something eternal.

In embracing our journey—immortal or not—we confront the ultimate question: What does it mean to live a life that feels immortally significant, yet is grounded in the fragility of the human experience? It's an ongoing dialogue between our finite presence and our longing for infinity, a narrative we're all crafting, one heartbeat at a time.

It's not the sheer number of years that will define our legacy, but the depth of our engagement with life in every breath we take. Whether we are to be ephemeral flames or enduring stars, let's ensure the light we cast is warm, vibrant, and forever inscribed in the hearts of those we touch.

Appendix A: Comprehensive Nutrition Guide for Longevity

Strolling through this high-velocity train of thought we call life, food becomes more than just fuel; it transforms into a code of sorts, one that can either program us for a stint or a saga. Diving into the warmth of a thought where we peek into the Pandora's Box named 'eternal life', nutrition is that low-hanging fruit, ripe for the picking yet so often overlooked.

What we put on our forks can be the silent narrators of our life's story, with the potential to add more pages, more chapters. Imagine that, the alchemy of it all, mixing and matching the humble plants, the wild catches, and the pastoral picks to give our cells a fighting chance to outrun the clock.

Nutrition Essentials for a Life More... Perpetual?

Sure, dipping our toes into the fountain of youth isn't as simple as munching on kale rather than candy, but it's a start. We've heard the buzzwords: antioxidants, polyphenols, omega-3s. They are keys to unlock doors we've accepted as walls. Fruits and berries, they're like little nuggets of life-preserving gold, while veggies stand as the sturdy, unyielding pillars holding up the temple that is our body.

Then there's the magic woven by nuts and seeds, and the tale goes that these little guys are brimming with secrets to keep the inner cogs well-oiled and turning with ease.

Lean proteins, whether from the land, the sea, or a leaf, whisper promises of renewal and repair—so crucial when dreaming of timelessness.

The Art of Balancing Macros and Micros

Carbs, proteins, fats—the triad that dances in harmony, when done right, can lead to an uproarious standing ovation from every cell in your body. It's not just about macronutrients though; those micronutrients are like a sprinkle of stardust on the canvas of our longevity. Zinc, magnesium, selenium—the names sound pulled from a celestial guidebook, each playing their part in an intricate cosmic dance.

Let's not get caught in the net of complication though. Balance isn't perfection; it's the art of ebbing and flowing with the natural rhythms of our bodies. It's choosing sweet potatoes over fries, not because you must, but because you're in tune with the melody of your well-being.

Foods That Fight the Clock

A true nomad of the nutritional desert wouldn't embark without the essentials. Here, we treasure foods tinted with the hue of health—leafy greens, cruciferous fighters like broccoli and cauliflower, and berries that punch above their weight in antioxidants. Turmeric, ginger, and green tea stand as the trinity of anti-inflammatory prowess, their soothing effect a balm for weary cells.

The age-defying puzzle isn't complete without good fats. Avocados, olive oil, and those fish that glide through pristine waters—they carry a secret in the form of omega-3 fatty acids. It's a love letter to your heart and brain in every bite.

It's almost poetic, the way fibers from whole grains and legumes escort toxins out, like bouncers ensuring the party inside our microbiome is exclusive to friendly guests. Did you ever think a humble bean could be a guardian of your gastrointestinal galaxy?

So, let's not obsess over the minutiae, but rather revel in the symphony of nutrient-dense foods, and allow instinct to sometimes take the wheel on this long, exhilarating ride towards what could be our personal brand of immortality. A feast for the cells, a toast to the passing of years, a nod to the fact that maybe, just maybe, we can nudge the sun to rise and set on our terms, ever so subtly.

Winding down this chapter, we carry with us the notion that what we eat is the whisper of life into our being. It's a gentle, yet resolute reminder that we're creatures not just meant to survive, but to flourish—and perhaps even to outlast the expectations etched by time itself.

Appendix B: Recommended Reading and Resources

We've journeyed through the labyrinthine pathways that might lead to the holy grail of immortality, grappling with concepts that dance on the edge of science fiction and philosophy, right? We've talked biology, technology, spirituality—you name it. But now, you might be yearning for more. It's like you've got this intellectual itch that only the most tantalizing reads can scratch, and you're in luck because I've assembled a treasure trove for the insatiably curious.

Let's kick things off with some foundational reads that'll give your brain that delightful blend of challenge and satisfaction. I mean, if you're looking to push the boundaries of your understanding—and I'm betting you are—these selected titles are prime material.

Science and Biology of Aging

- *The Telomere Effect* - Delve deep into the world of chromosomes and discover how tiny caps at the end of our DNA strands have massive implications for our health and longevity.

- *Lifespan: Why We Age—and Why We Don't Have To* - A groundbreaking exploration of the aging process and provocatively promising approaches that might just disrupt the very notion of growing old.

Health and Wellness

1. *How Not to Die* - Fusing medical insight with nutrition, this one rights the wrongs of modern diets and shines the light on foods that could add years to your life.

2. *Atomic Habits* - Get hooked on the tiny changes that breed monumental results, reshaping your behaviors to forge a robust, enduring you.

Philosophy and Spirituality

- *The Immortalists* - Philosophy married with storytelling, this one tugs at the threads of what it means to live knowing you could live forever.

- *The Book of Joy* - Perhaps immortality is worthless without joy, and here's a tome that unearths this timeless emotion in the face of life's highs and lows.

Technology and Futurism

1. *The Singularity is Near* - Buckle—no, don't buckle—just dive in! This read challenges your perceptions of technology, its trajectory, and its ultimate union with our biological fabric.

2. *Life 3.0: Being Human in the Age of Artificial Intelligence* - It's about AI, but more so, it's about us, humans, steering the ship into new, immortal sunrises.

But, hey, books aren't the only resources out there. Podcasts, documentaries, seminars—those can be your gateways to alternate perspectives and the latest thought waves crashing against the shore of collective consciousness. Look up seminars on integrative medicine, brush against the digital consciousness in webinars, fetch insights from biohacking podcasts, and let documentaries chronicle the successes (and failures) of those who dare to chase eternity.

Keep this list handy. Digest it slowly or binge it if that's your tempo. Either way, they say knowledge is immortal. So, as you feed your mind with these curated picks, remember that each idea learned, each paradigm shifted, and each habit formed can echo through your own slice of infinity.

Glossary of Key Terms and Concepts

Before we dive deeper into the immersive wonderland of extending our stay on this spinning rock, let's shake hands with some terms you'll bump into along the way. These are the breadcrumbs that'll help you navigate the dense forest of everlasting life—a pocket full of wisdom nuggets that aren't just fancy jargon but the ABCs of cheating the final curtain call.

Aging

Aging: It's the ticking clock, the biological countdown that's more relentless than your morning alarm. It's what turns sprightly teens into wise old-timers. At its core, it's the gradual loss of the body's oomph, which, to no surprise, catches up with us all.

Antioxidants

Antioxidants: These are the Luke Skywalkers in your body's galaxy, fighting off the Darth Vader of molecules—free radicals. They're the good guys that put up one heck of a fight to keep you looking more like a fresh spring chicken rather than a worn-out leather bag.

Biotechnology

Biotechnology: Think of biotech as that friend who's really into crafting, but instead of making friendship bracelets, they're redesigning the very fabric of life. It's the playground where science meets nature to tinker with the building blocks of existence.

Caloric Restriction

Caloric Restriction: Let's talk about dieting, but not just shaving off a few pounds for beach season. It's about eating less to trick your body into thinking you're a hunter-gatherer, boosting your lifespan as if hitting a high score in an arcade game.

Cellular Senescence

Cellular Senescence: It's like those cells decided to retire early but forgot to leave the office. These cells just hang around, not really working, and start gossiping toxins that are no good for their youthful neighbors still hustling away.

Consciousness Uploading

Consciousness Uploading: Ever thought of living inside a computer? Well, that's the sci-fi dream right here— beaming your mind into the digital realm to flick off the mortality switch. Tron, anyone?

Cryonics

Cryonics: That's the chilly idea of playing possum at sub-zero temperatures after you've passed, hoping the future has a thaw-and-revive solution. It's like putting leftovers in the freezer, but you're the leftovers, and the future is dinner time.

Genetic Engineering

Genetic Engineering: Armed with the latest and greatest in molecular scissors, scientists are in the lab, playing the ultimate game of Operation, snipping and saving the bits of DNA that might just hold the key to turning off the aging tap.

Longevity

Longevity: It's the measure of your life's runway. Some have a long strip, others have a short one, but either way, it's about how to add more tarmac to that strip, so you have loads of time before you need to lift off.

Meditation

Meditation: You could call it mind-gardening—a bit of inward focus, a dollop of breathing, and voila! You're tilling the soil of your noggin, planting seeds of zen, and growing a bumper crop of inner peace—on the house!

Regenerative Medicine

Regenerative Medicine: Doctors with a green thumb for human parts are the stars here, convincing your body to fix itself, grow new bits, or patching it up with lab-grown spares. It's like human body shop, except with a little more science and a lot more future.

Sirtuins

Sirtuins: Picture a tiny squad of proteins moonlighting as handymen, tightening the bolts and fixing the leaks in your cells. They're part of the reason Grandma's still rocking out after all these years, giving Father Time a run for his money.

Stem Cells

Stem Cells: The renaissance artists of the cell world, these versatile little blobs of potential can become anything—the brain, bone, or heart cells—whatever you need, they're up for the task. Handy little chaps, wouldn't you say?

Transhumanism

Transhumanism: This is the buffet of ideologies that says, "You know what? Being human is cool, but what if we could be more?" It's about buffing our stats with tech and science to leapfrog right over Mother Nature's head.

Keep this glossary close; it's your toolkit, your cheat sheet. As we keep trekking, these terms will light up the path. Keep a tab on them; they're the touchstones of our juicy jamboree into the land where 'forever' isn't just a pipe dream, it's a pillar of the itinerary.